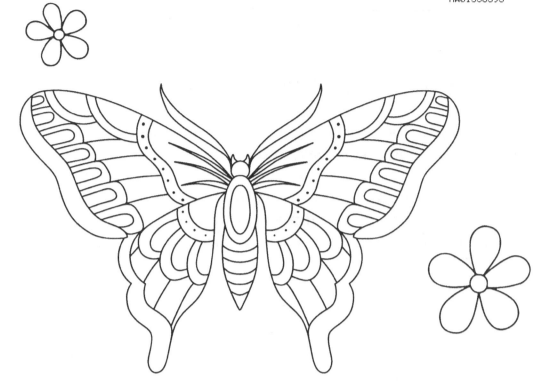

This Book Belongs to

_____

_____

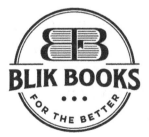

HAPPY AND EASY COLORING BOOK

Large Prints COLORING BOOK for Adults

2024 Copyright BLIKBOOKS

ALL RIGHTS RESERVED

The Power of Color

"Color is a power which directly influences the soul." - Wassily Kandinsky.

This book is not just about coloring, it's about the power of colors and how they can transform your mood, your day, and even your life.

Think about it. The bright yellow of a sunflower can instantly lift your spirits. The deep blue of the ocean can calm your mind. The vibrant red of a rose can ignite passion in your heart. Colors have an undeniable impact on our emotions and well-being.

In this book, you'll find 40 unique designs created by a professional artist. These designs range from animals to winter landscapes, from food to flowers, and so much more. Each design is easy to color with alternating thick and thin lines for different levels of challenge.

Coloring isn't just for kids anymore. It's a powerful tool for relaxation and stress relief for people of all ages!

You'll also find tips and techniques on how to use markers or pencils, along with suggestions for nice combinations of colors. These practical tips will help you make the most out of your coloring experience.

The pages are single-sided to reduce the bleed-through problem found in some other coloring books.

But this book isn't just about coloring; it's also about inspiration. In this book, you'll find inspiring quotes that will boost your happiness and self-esteem.

So grab your favourite set of colors and let them work their magic on these pages. Let each stroke fill you with joy, peace, and tranquility.

Remember, there are no rules when it comes to coloring. It's all about expressing yourself freely and letting your creativity flow.

ENJOY EVERY MOMENT!

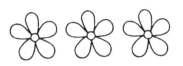

Why coloring is good for all of us!

Scientific studies have shown that coloring can be a therapeutic activity for people of all ages, including beginners and seniors.

Coloring and Mental Health: A study published in the Journal of the American Art Therapy Association found that just 30 minutes of structured coloring can lead to significant reductions in anxiety and improved mood. This suggests that coloring can be a cost-effective and accessible tool to help manage mental health issues.

Coloring and Dementia: A study in the Journal of Geriatric Psychiatry and Neurology found that art therapy, including coloring, can help improve the quality of life for people with dementia. It can help to reduce symptoms such as agitation and depression, and improve communication and social interaction.

Coloring and Depression: A study in the Journal of Affective Disorders found that art therapy, including coloring, can be an effective treatment for depression. The researchers found that participants who engaged in art therapy reported significant reductions in symptoms of depression and improved quality of life.

Interesting Facts

Coloring can help to induce a state of mindfulness and reduce stress. When you're coloring, you're focused on the task at hand and not on your worries or anxieties.

Coloring can help to improve motor skills and vision. The act of coloring requires coordination between the brain, the eyes, and the hands, which can help to improve fine motor skills.

Coloring can help to improve focus and concentration. It requires attention to detail and concentration, which can help to improve these skills in other areas of life.

Coloring can help to improve creativity. It allows for self-expression and the opportunity to experiment with different colors and designs.

Coloring can be a social activity. Coloring groups and clubs have popped up all over the world, providing a space for people to come together, relax, and enjoy the benefits of colouring.

Coloring stimulates several different areas of the brain related to motor skills, senses, creativity, and the 'reward pathway'. This not only enhances cognitive functioning but also promotes feelings of satisfaction and accomplishment when completing a picture - making it an excellent activity for people living with dementia or Alzheimer's disease.

Full Citations:
1. Curry, N. A., & Kasser, T. (2005). Can coloring mandalas reduce anxiety? Art Therapy, 22(2), 81-85.
2. Rusted, J., Sheppard, L., & Waller, D. (2006). A multi-centre randomized control group trial on the use of art therapy for older people with dementia. Group Analysis, 39(4), 517-536. 3. Monti, D. A., Peterson, C., Kunkel, E. J., Hauck, W. W., Pequignot, E., Rhodes, L., & Brainard, G. C. (2006). A randomized, controlled trial of mindfulness-based art therapy (MBAT) for women with cancer. Psycho-Oncology: Journal of the Psychological, Social and Behavioral Dimensions of Cancer, 15(5), 363-373

Tips & Techniques

1. Choosing the Right Tools: According to art therapists, colored pencils are often recommended for beginners because they allow for great precision and control. On the other hand, markers provide vibrant colors but may bleed through pages if not used carefully.

2. Preventing Bleed Through: To prevent marker ink from bleeding onto the next page, place an extra sheet of paper or cardstock between pages while coloring. This will absorb any excess ink.

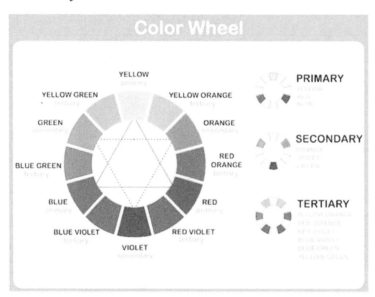

3. Combining Colors:

A study published in the Journal of Experimental Psychology found that humans naturally prefer certain color combinations over others because of how our brains process visual information.

Basic color theory

- Complementary colors (colors opposite each other on the color wheel) create high contrast and stand out when used together.
- Analogous colors (colors next to each other on the color wheel) create harmonious blends.

4. Experimentation is Key: Don't be afraid to experiment with different types of markers or pencils until you find what works best for you. As per industry experts like Johanna Basford - a pioneer in adult coloring books - "The key is just to get started... pick up a pencil or pen and make your mark."

5. Take Your Time: Coloring isn't about rushing towards completion; it's about enjoying the process itself which has been proven by research at Harvard Medical School showing that mindful activities like coloring can induce relaxation response in body thus reducing stress levels.

COLOR TEST

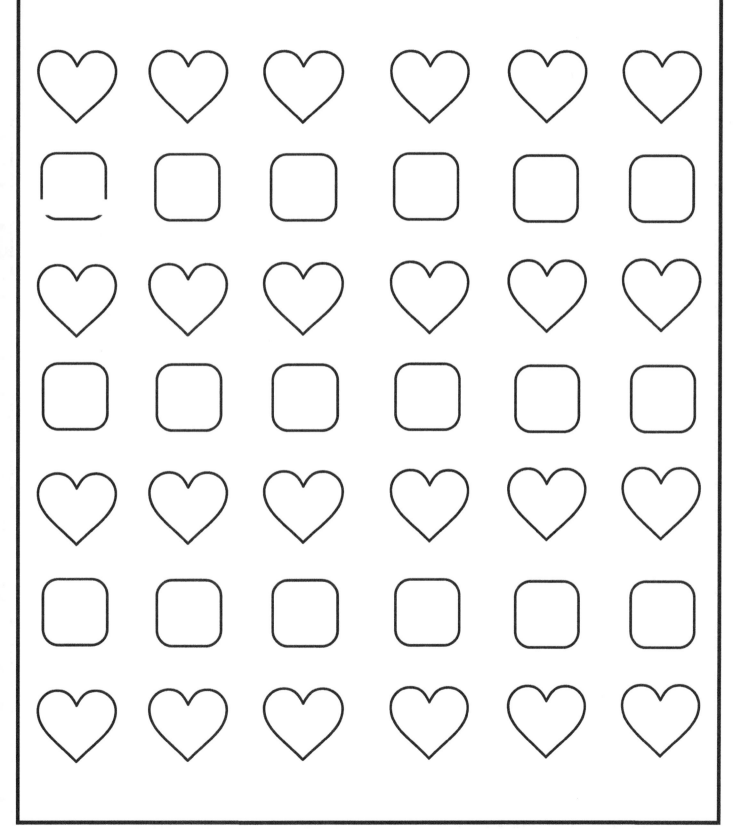

COLOR TEST

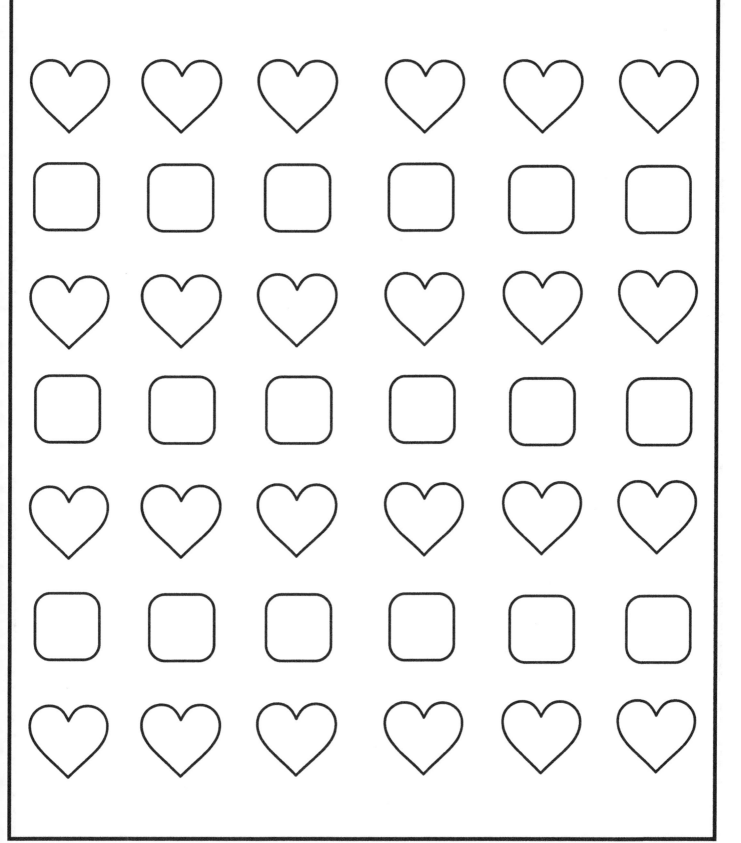

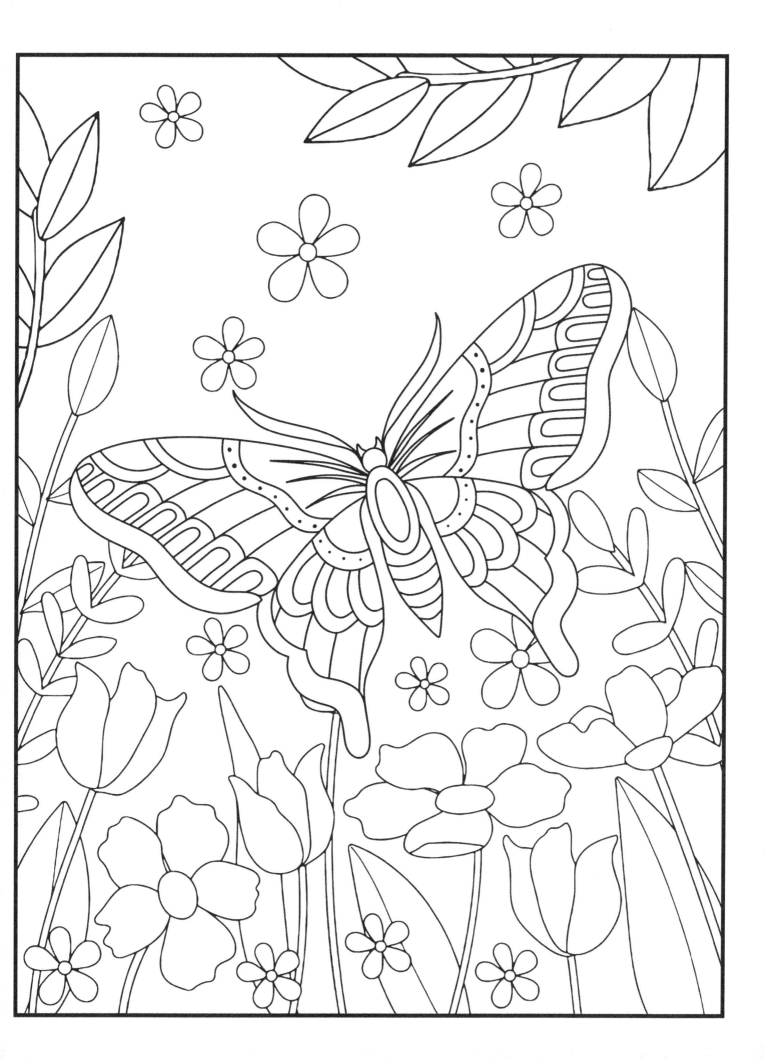

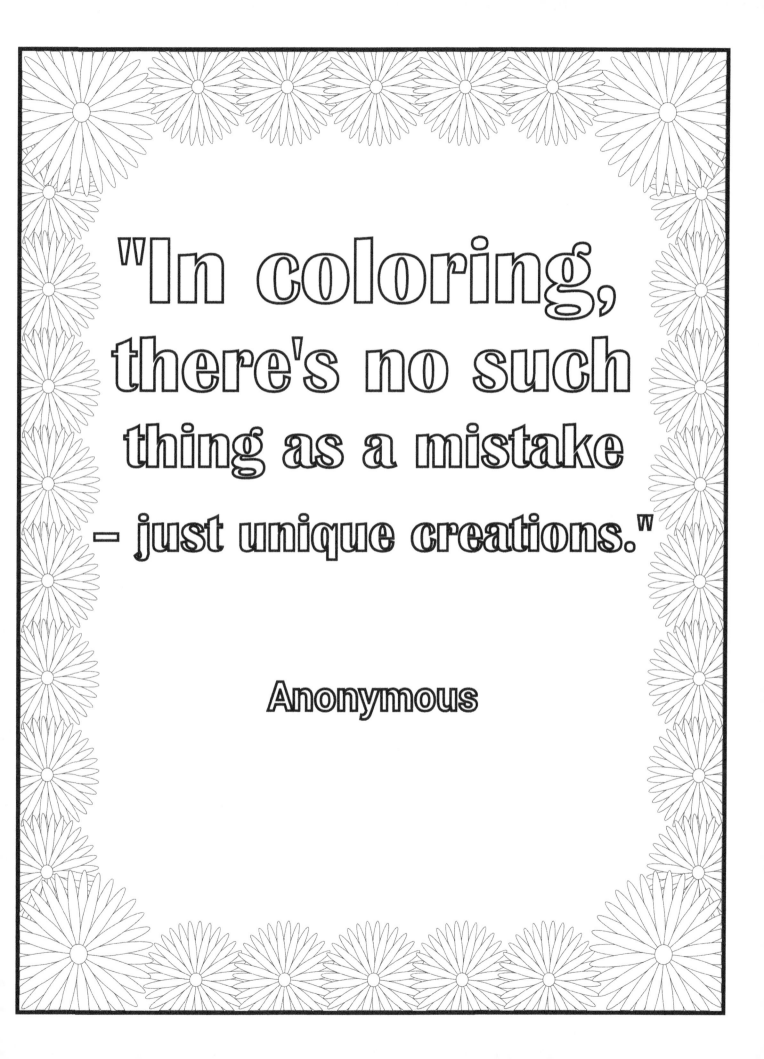

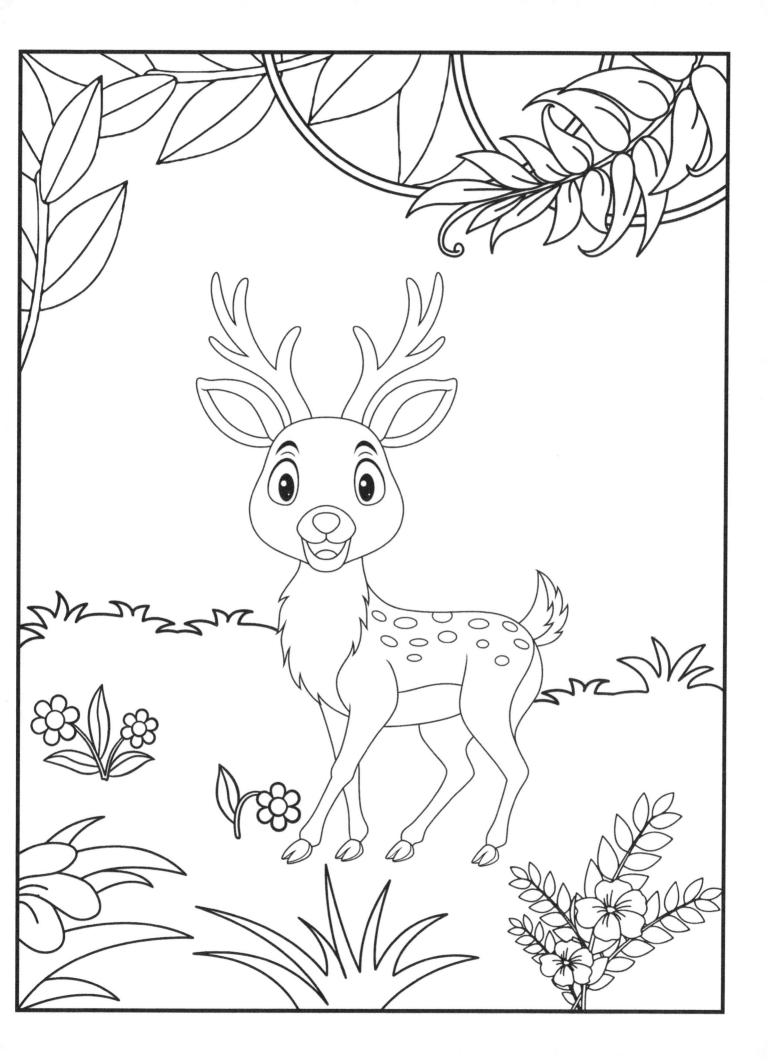

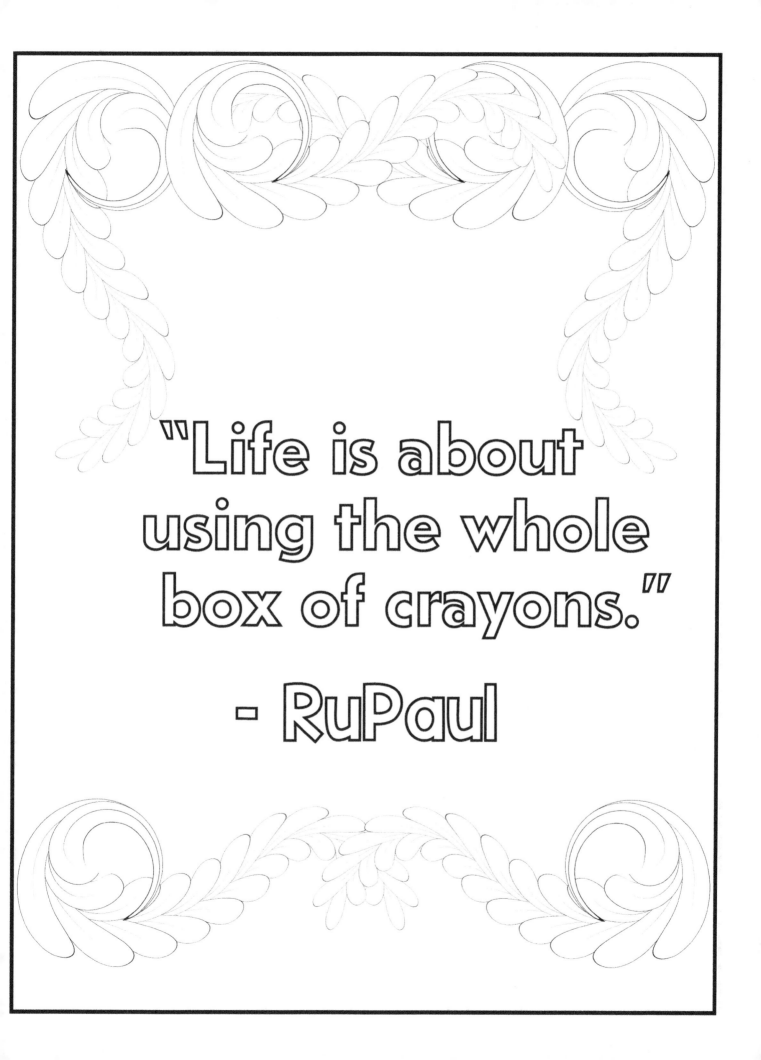

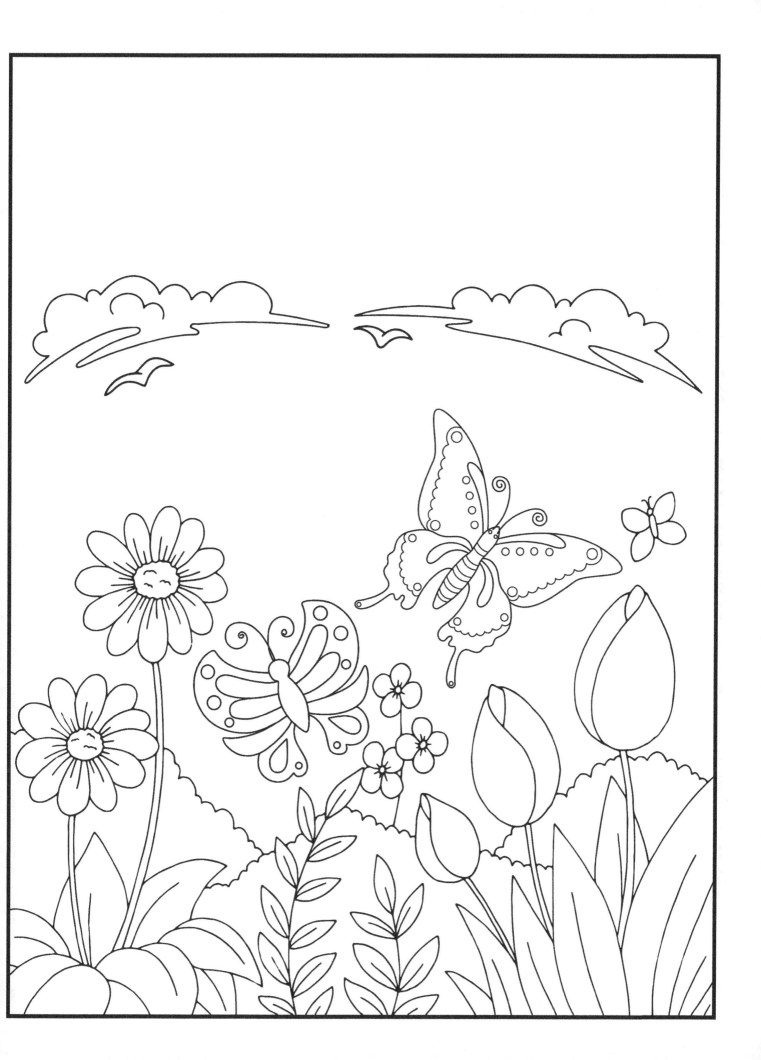

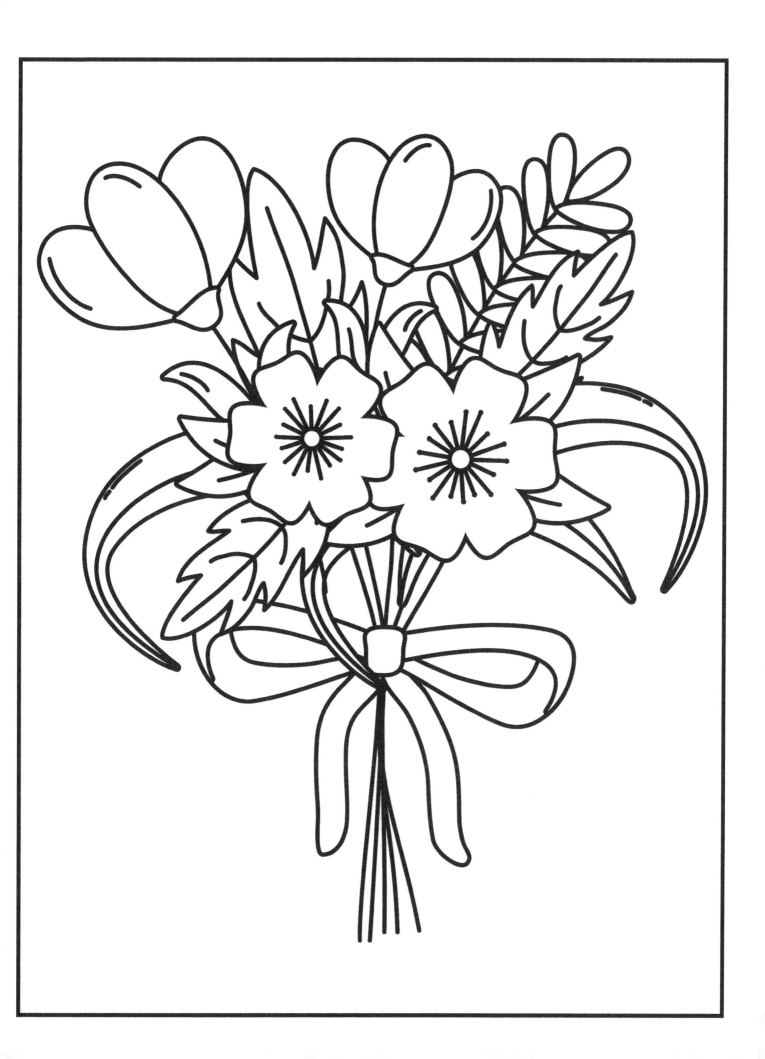

"COLORING OUTSIDE
THE LINES IS
A FINE ART."

- Kim Nance

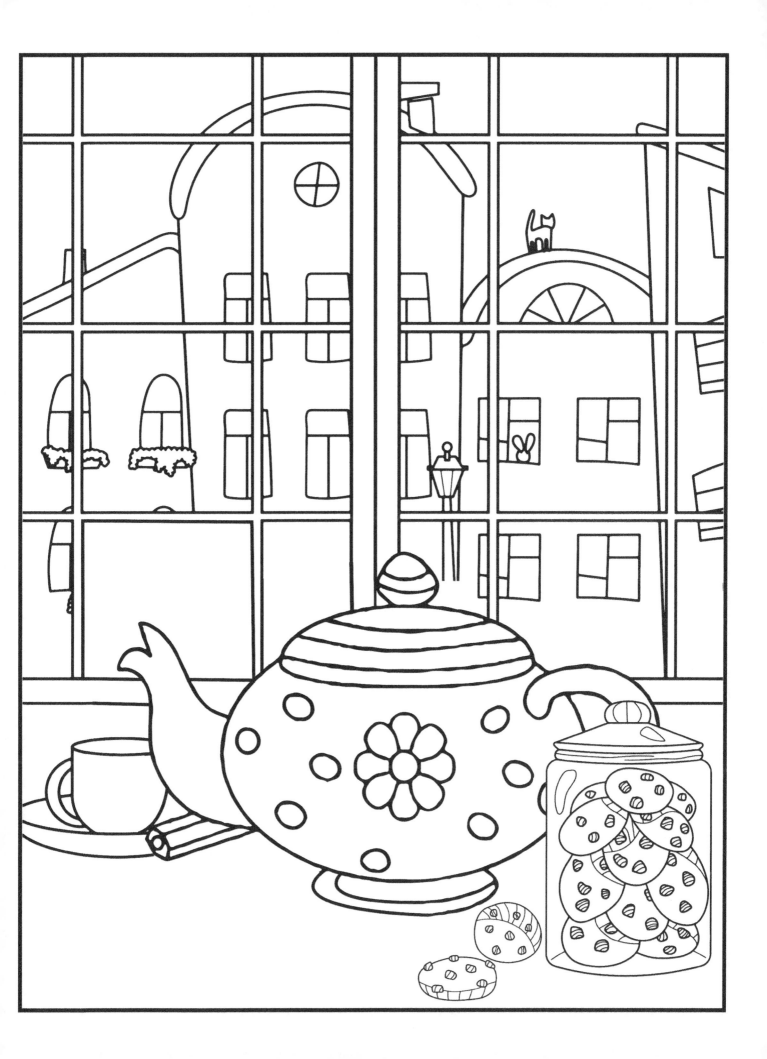

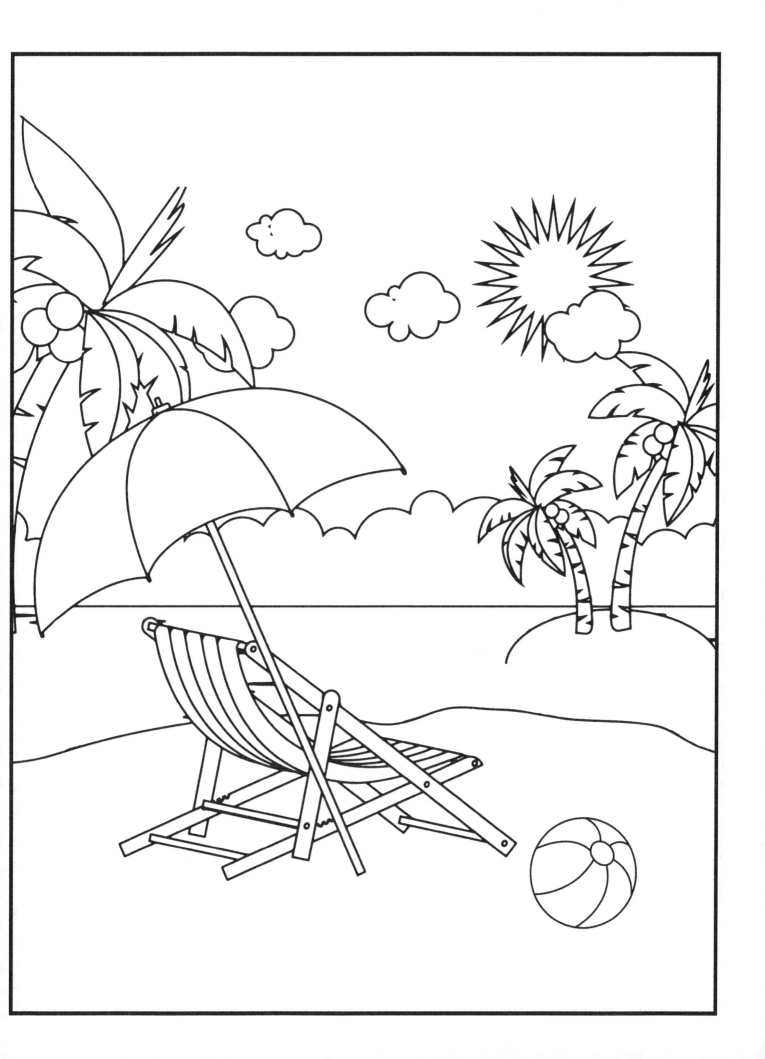

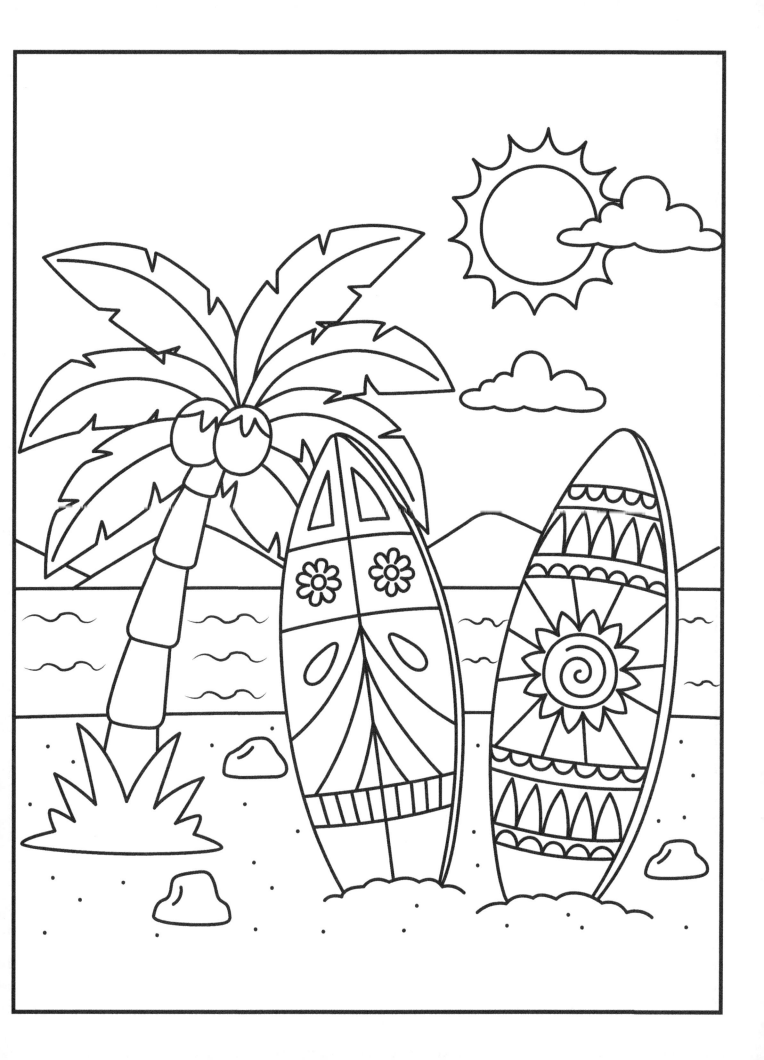

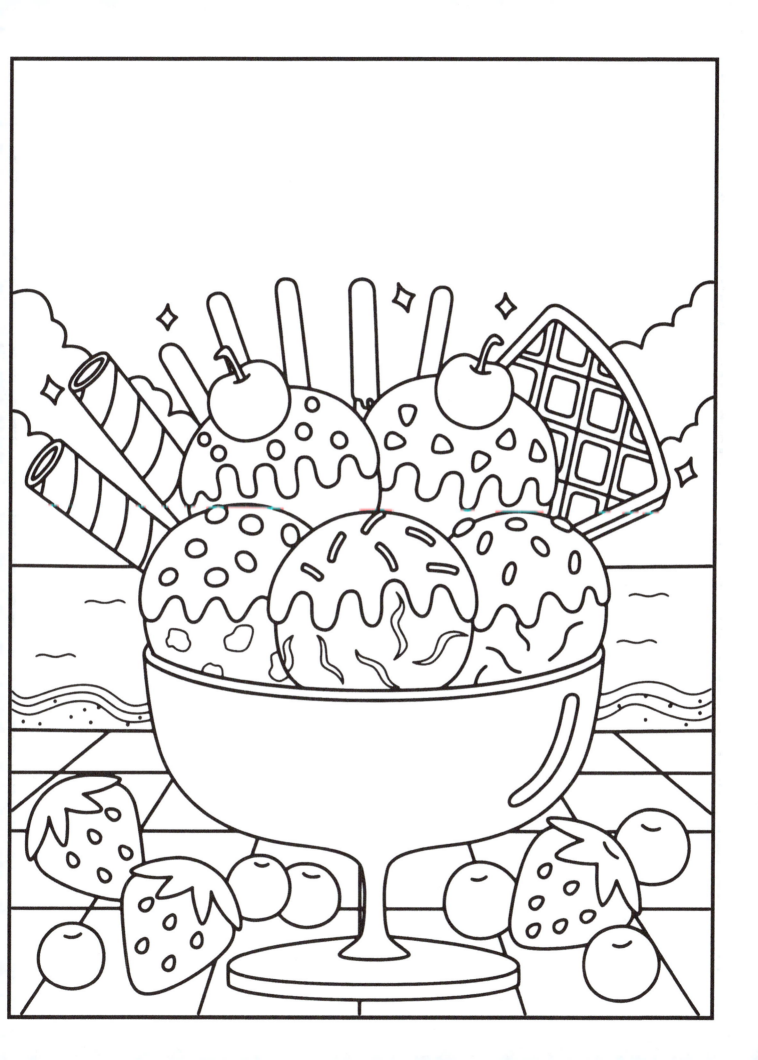

"Colour in a picture is like enthusiasm in life"

- Vincent Van Gogh

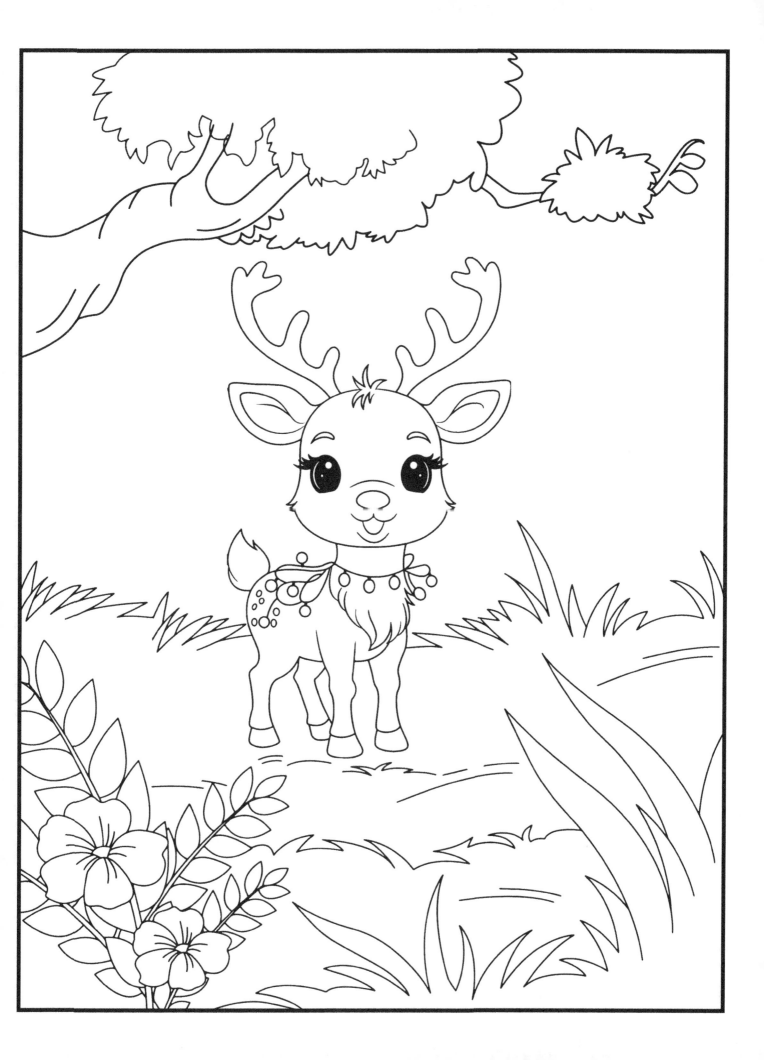

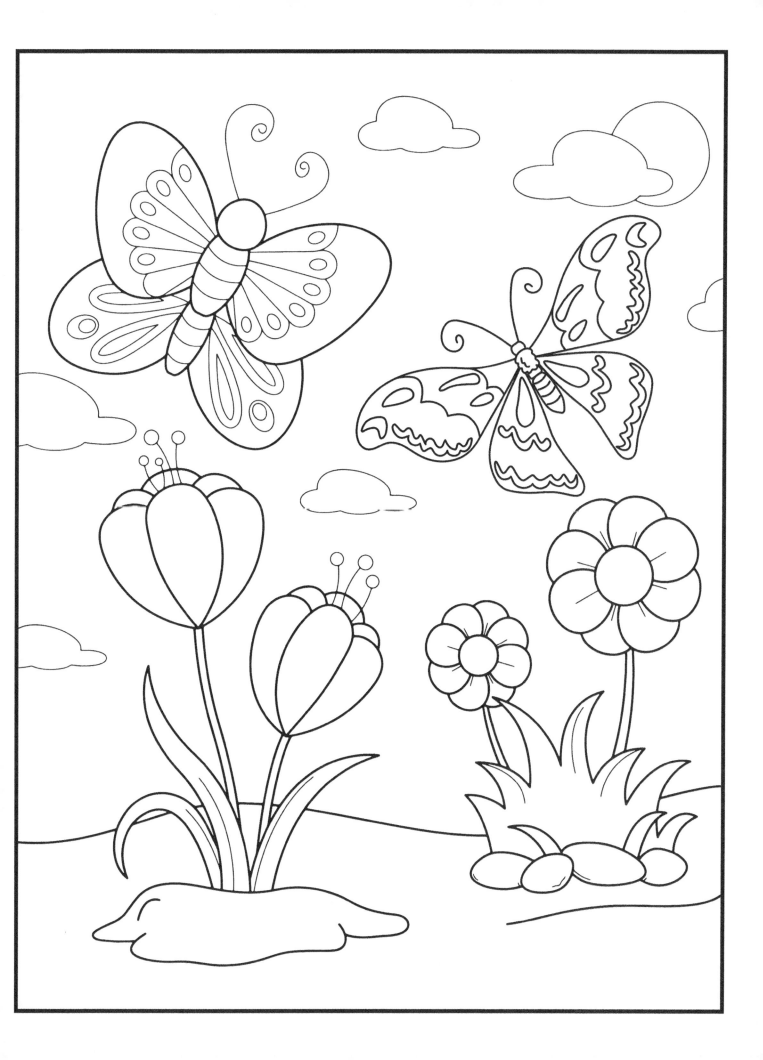

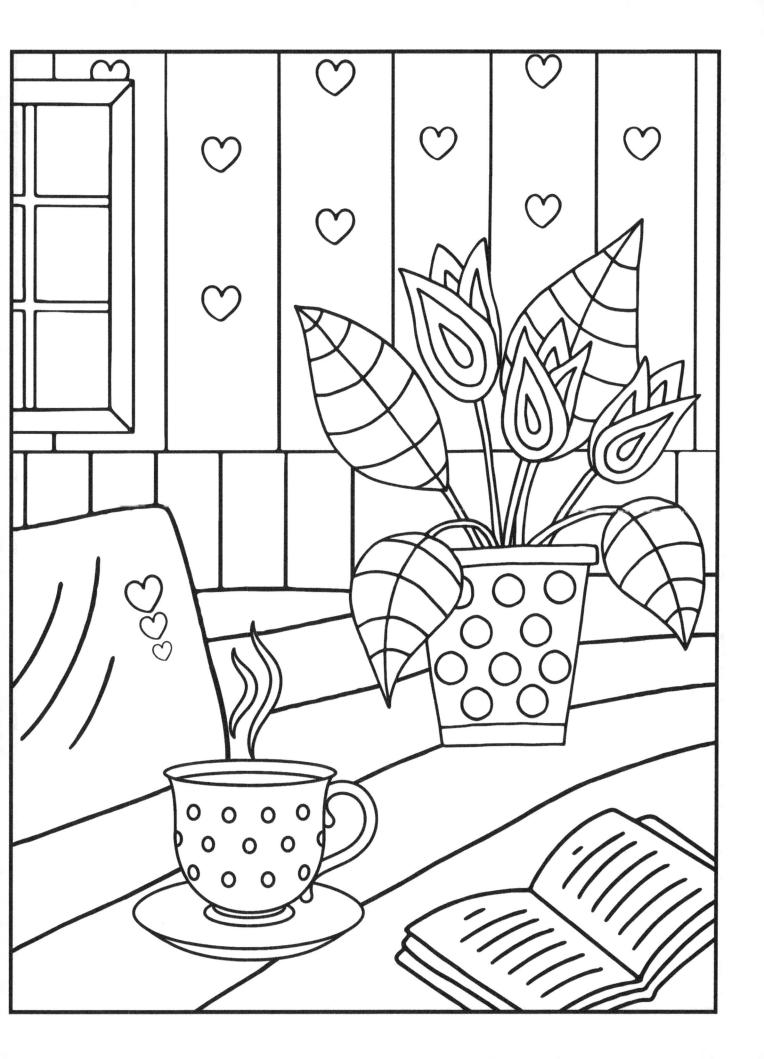

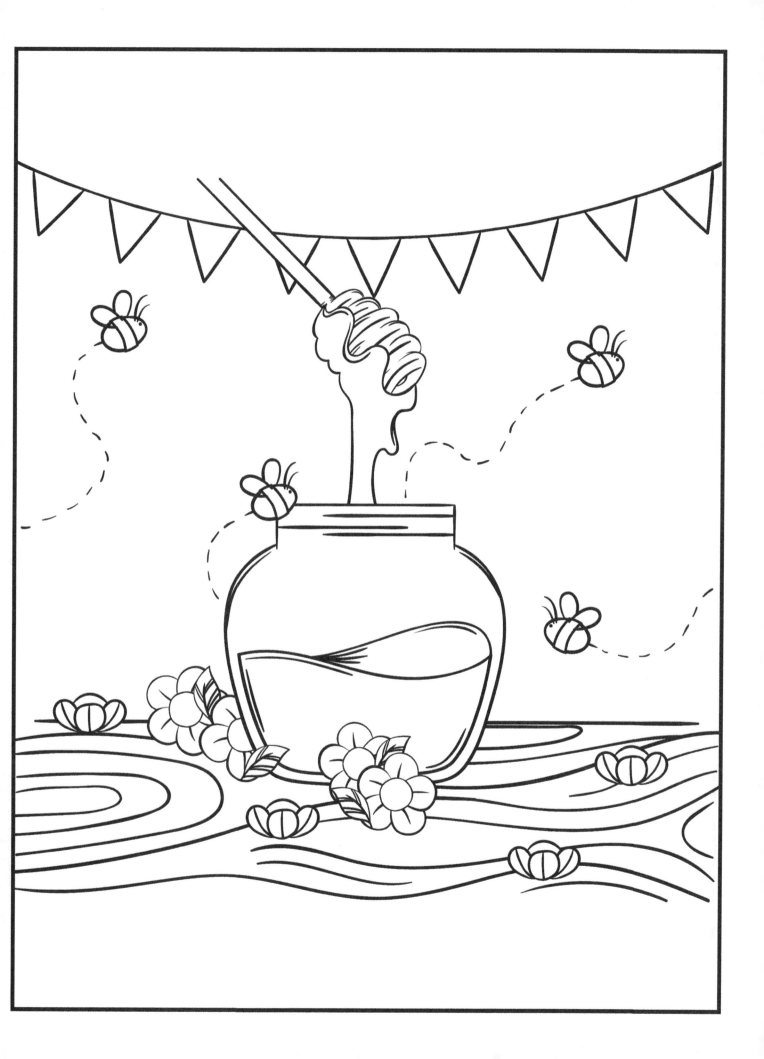

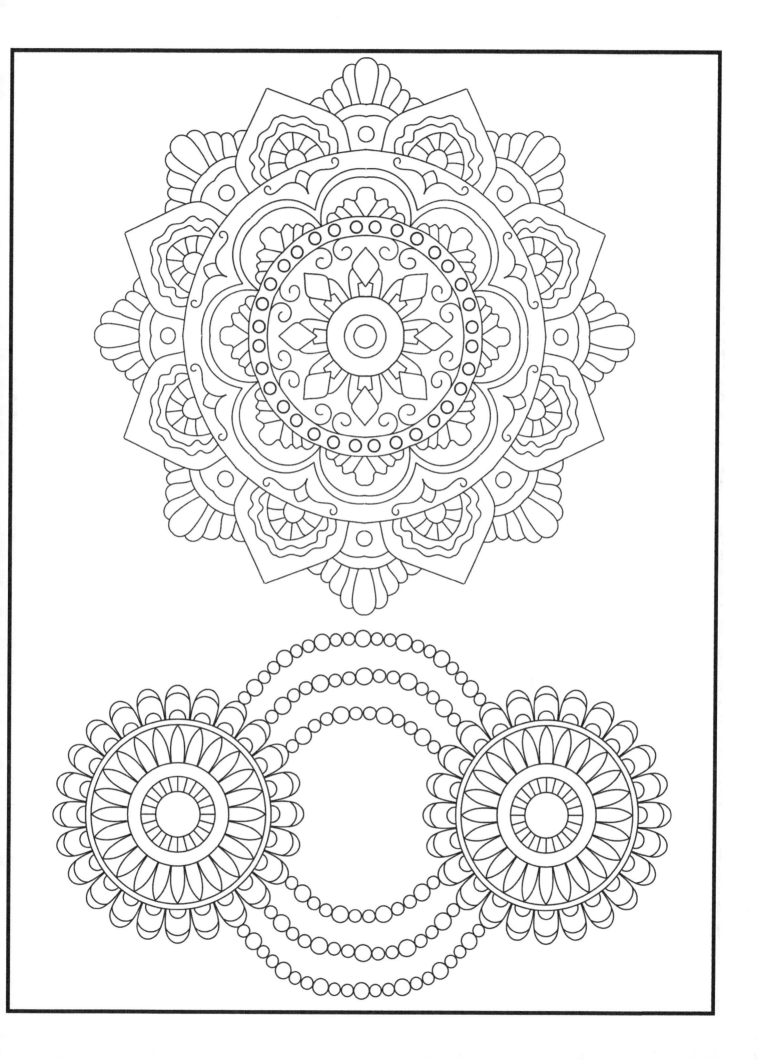

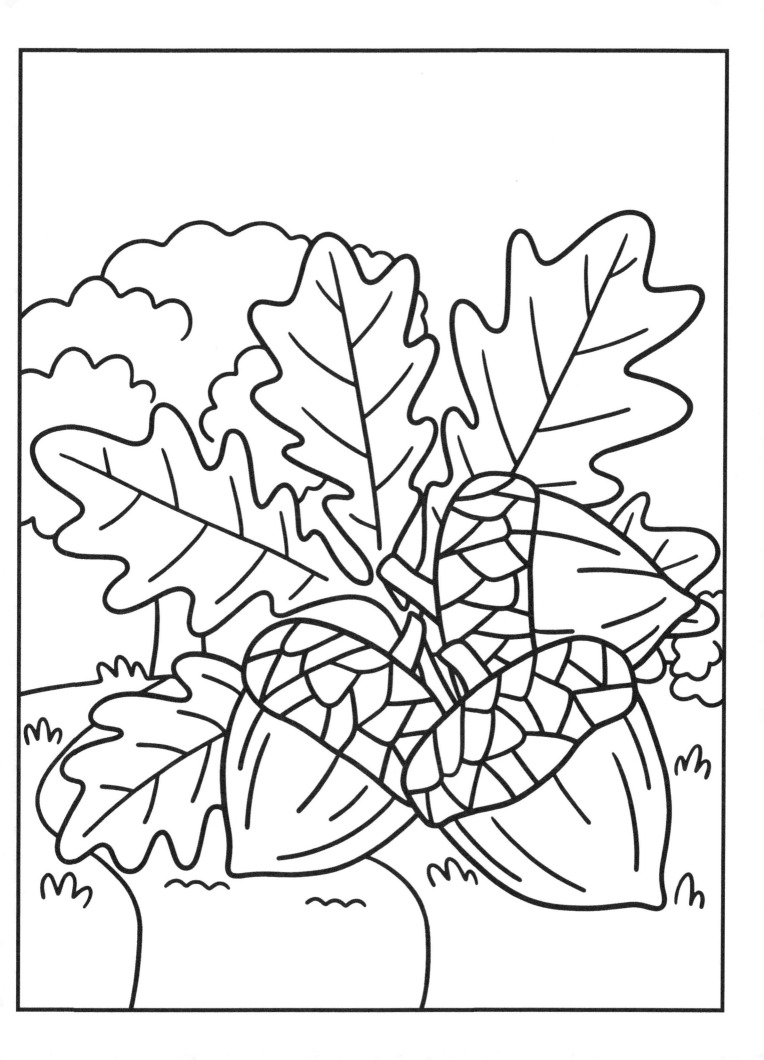

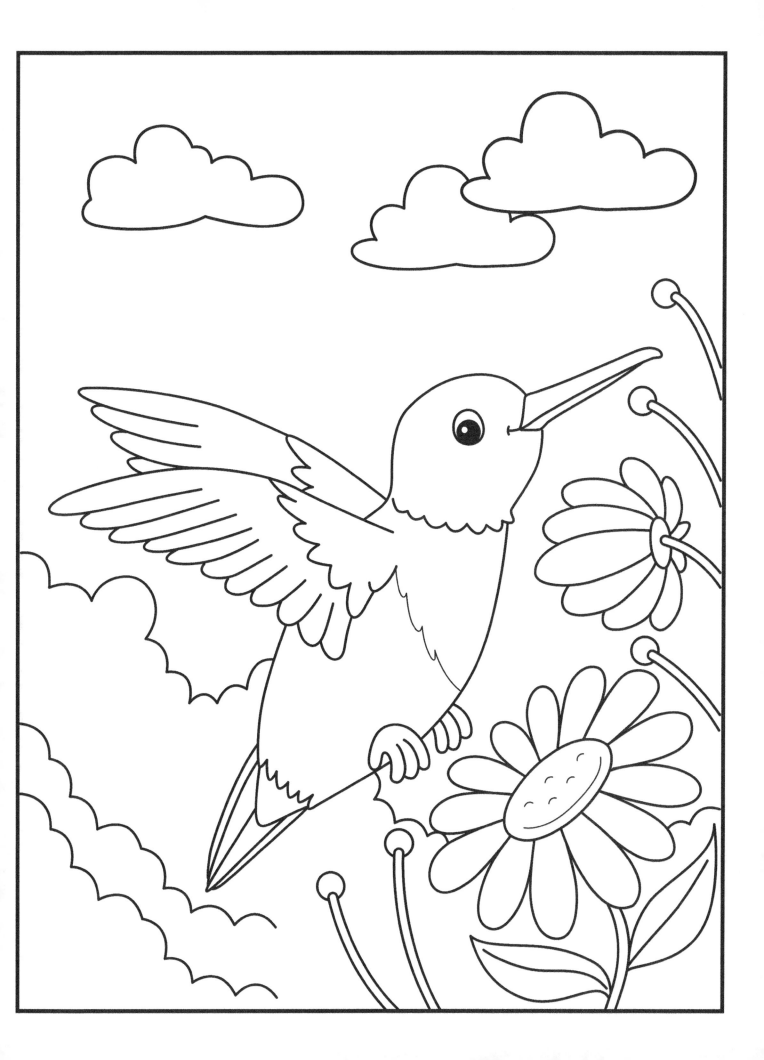

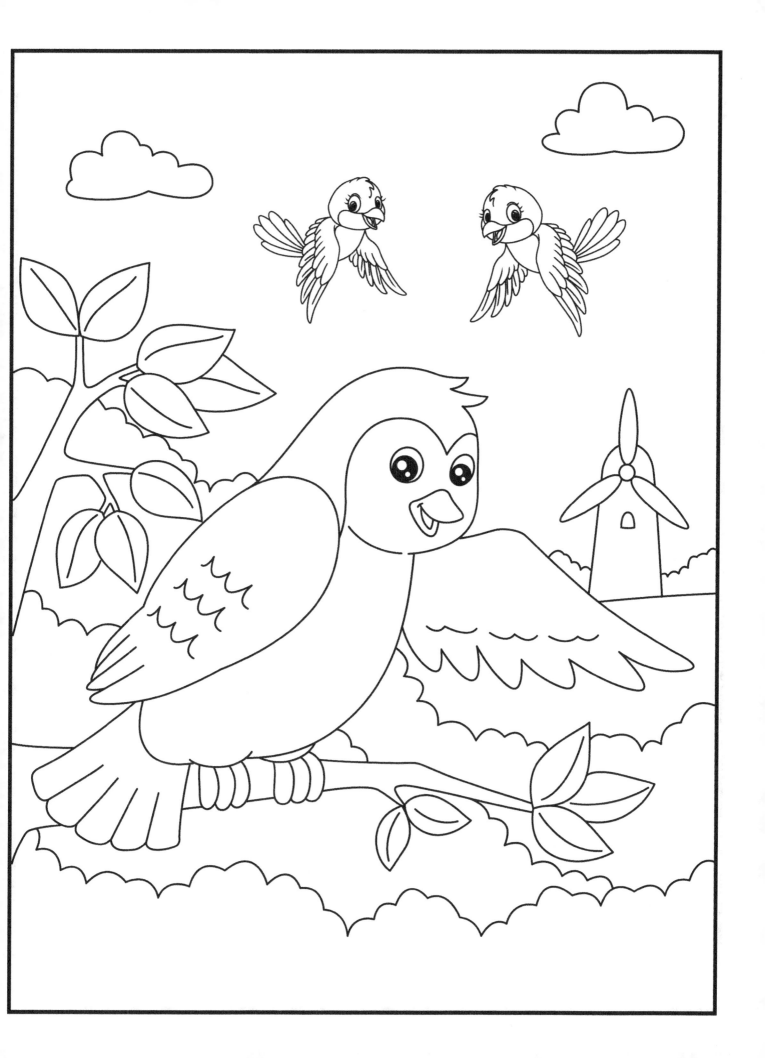

"Colors speak louder than words."

- Anonymous

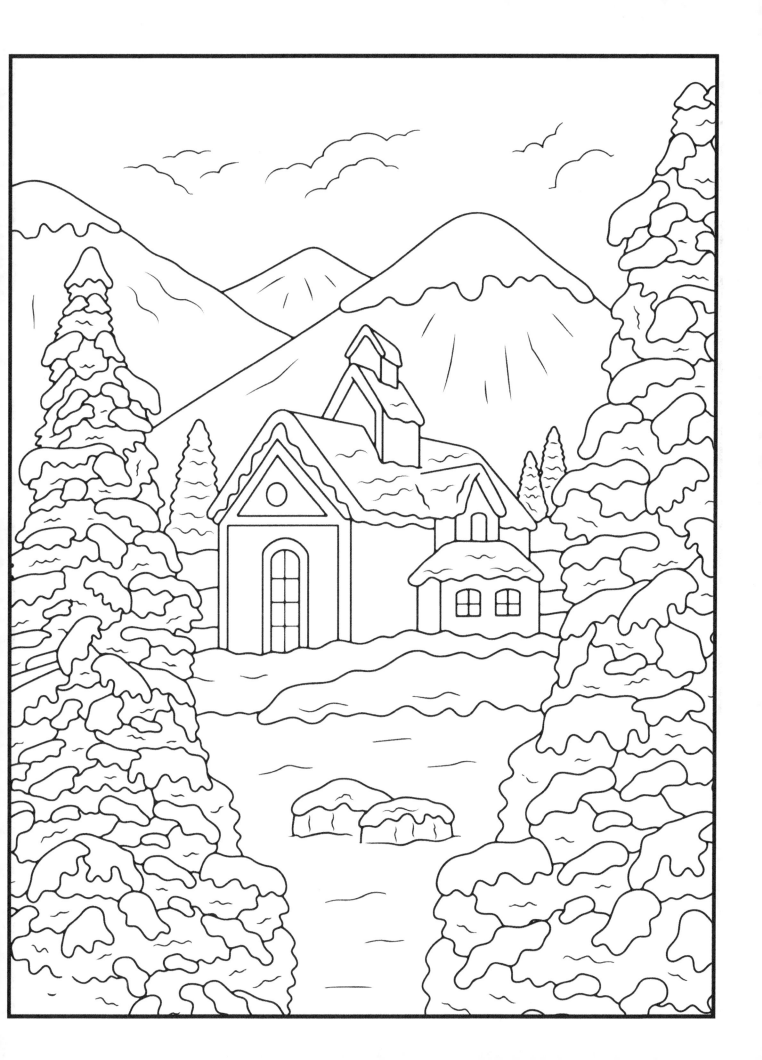

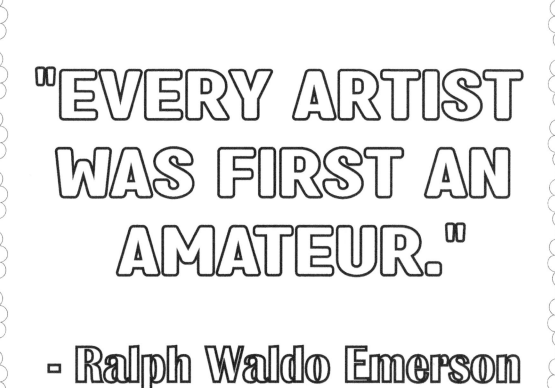

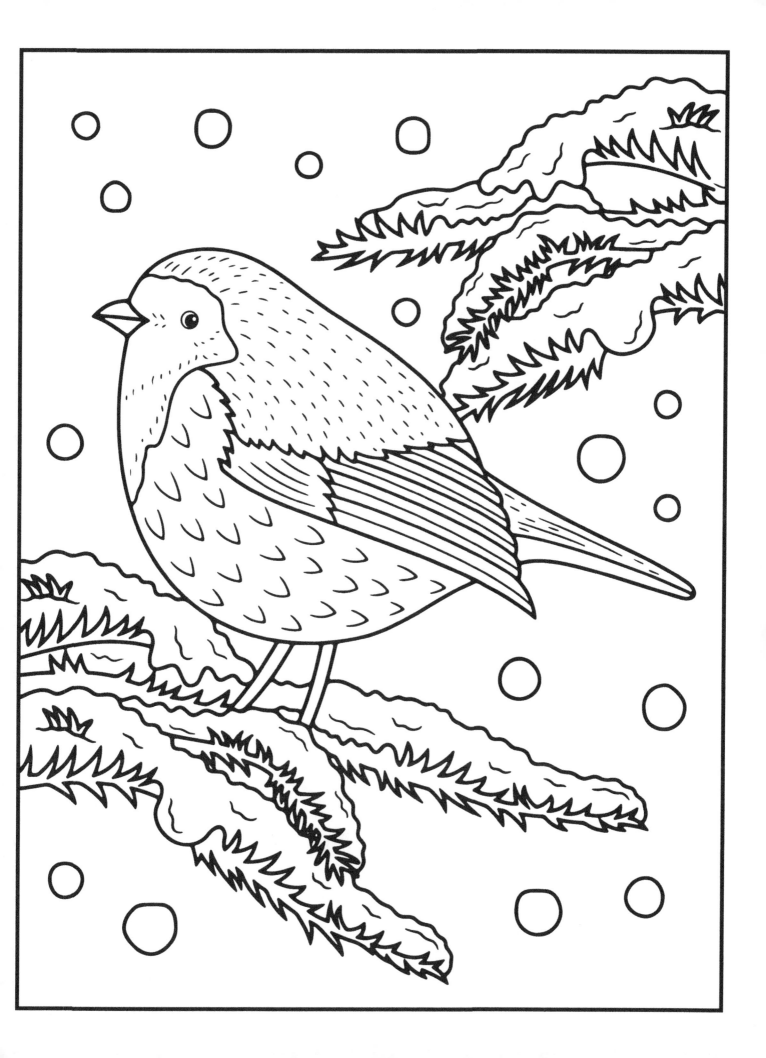

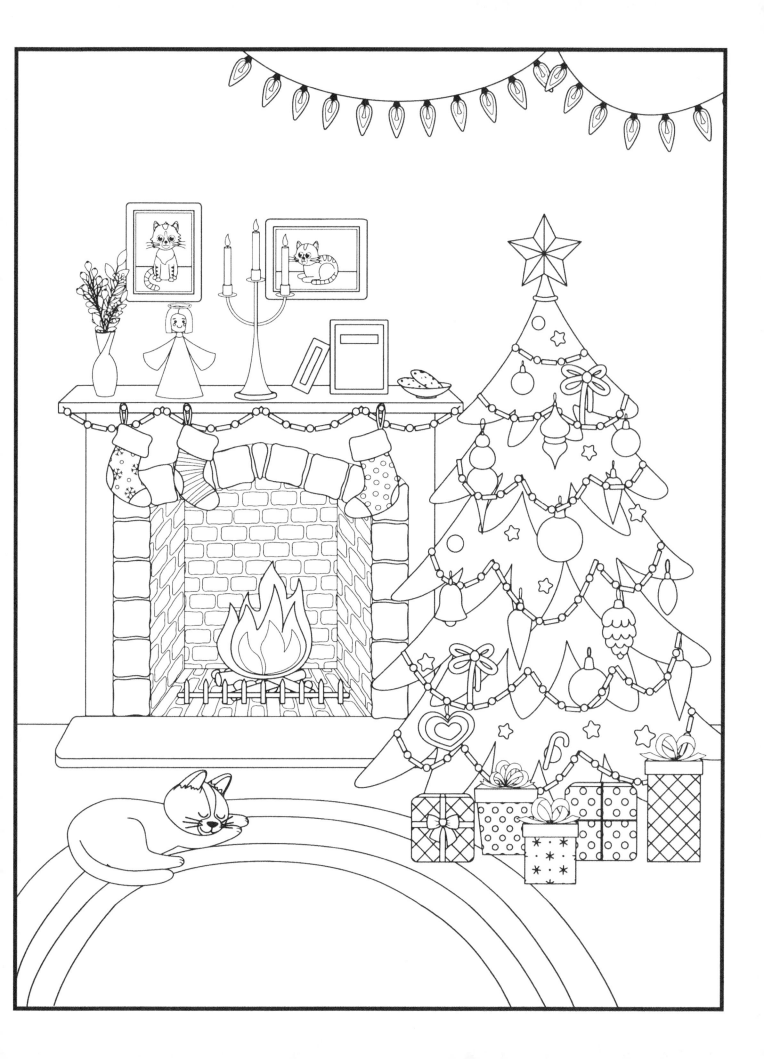

"Creativity takes courage."

- Henri Matisse

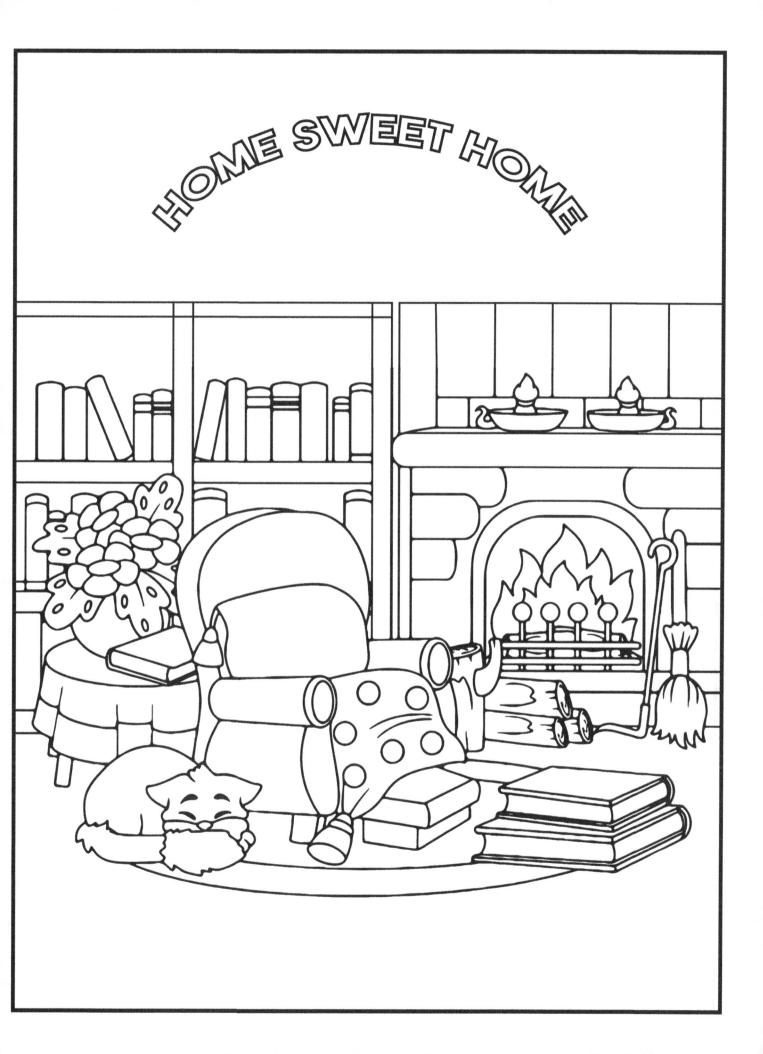

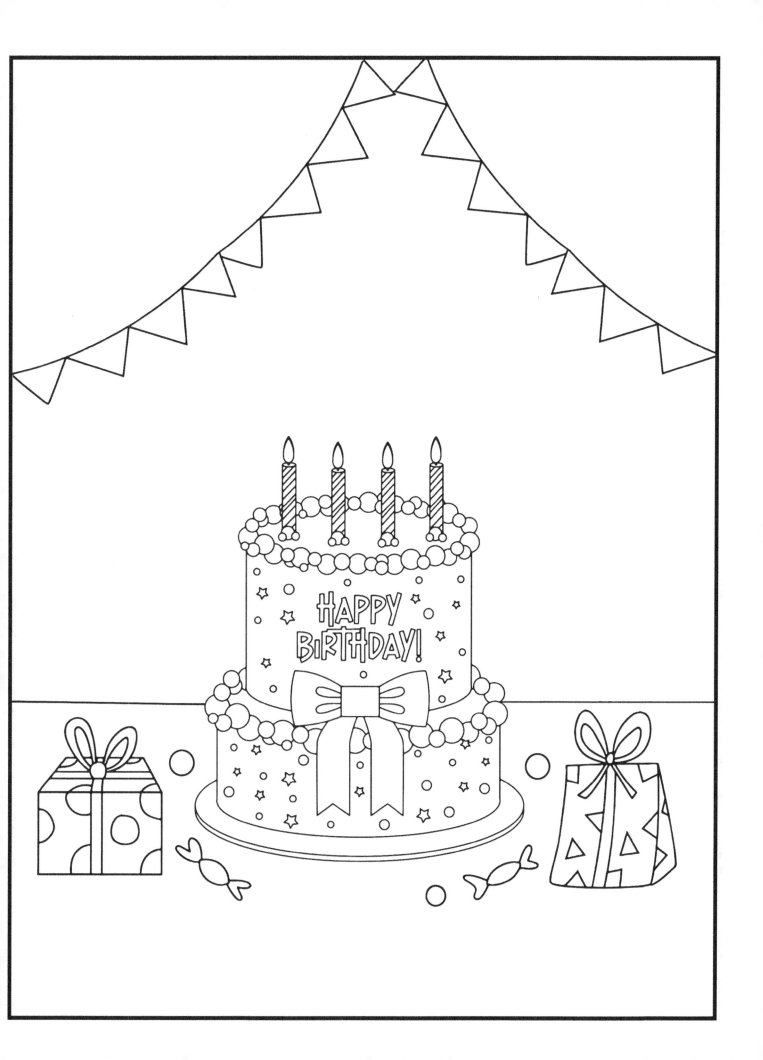

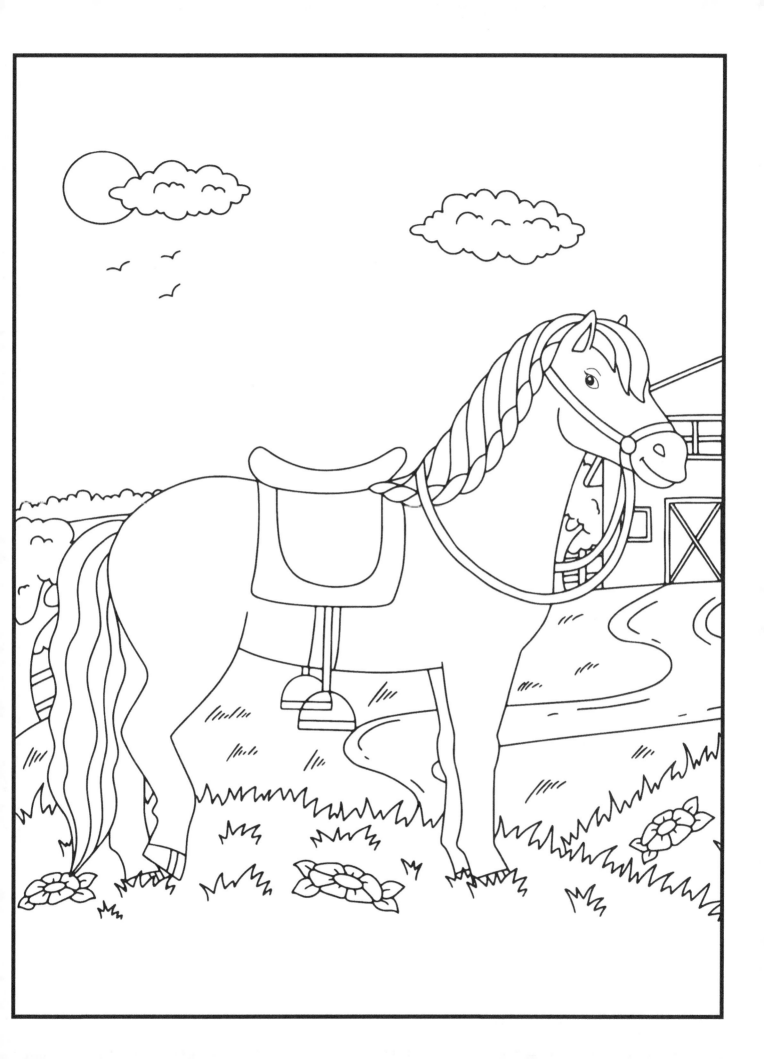

"In our hectic lives,
color can be an
escape to tranquility
and personal expression."

- Anonymous

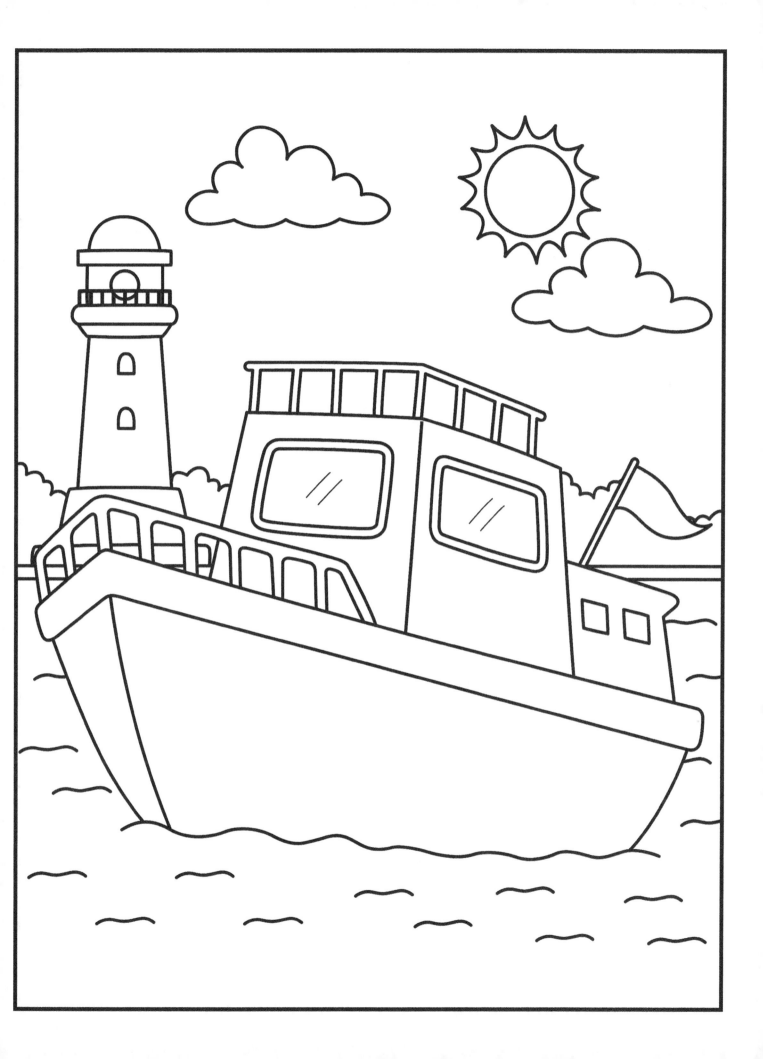

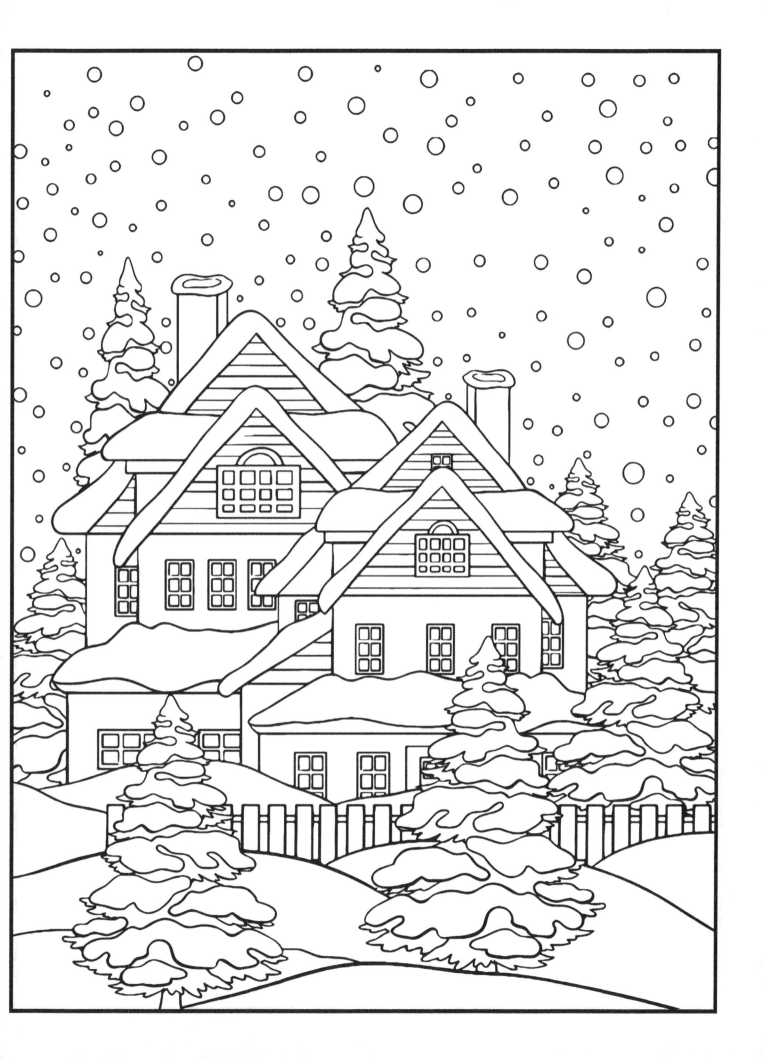

"An artist cannot fail; it's a success to be one"

- Charles Horton Cooley

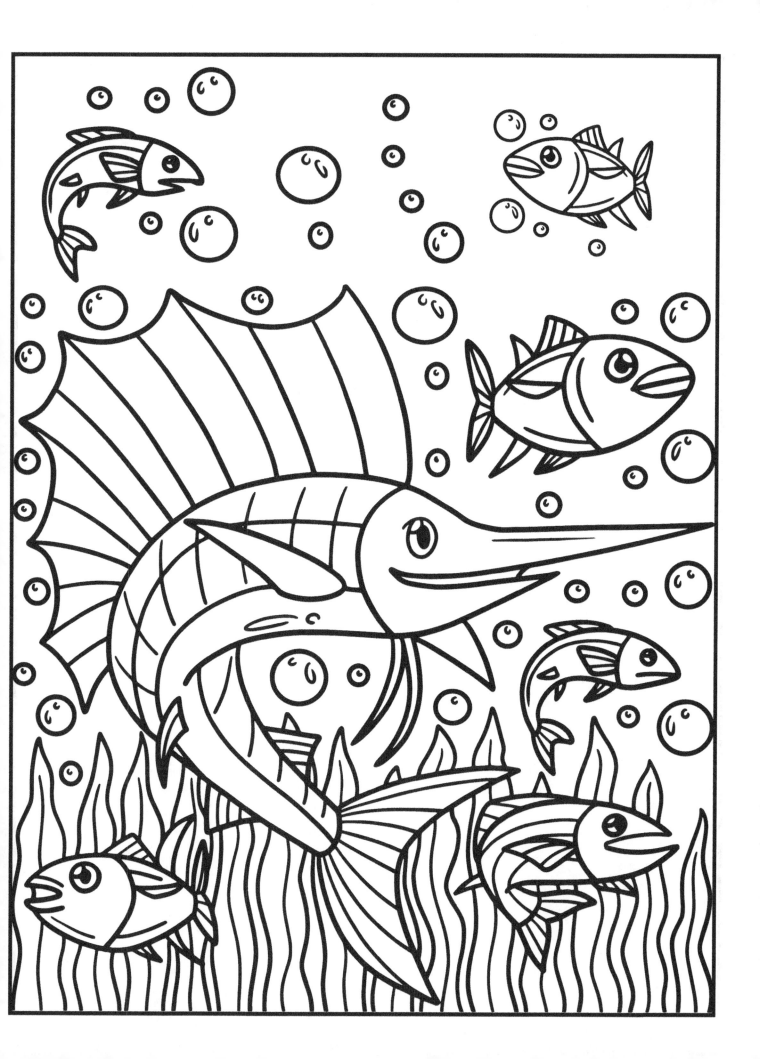

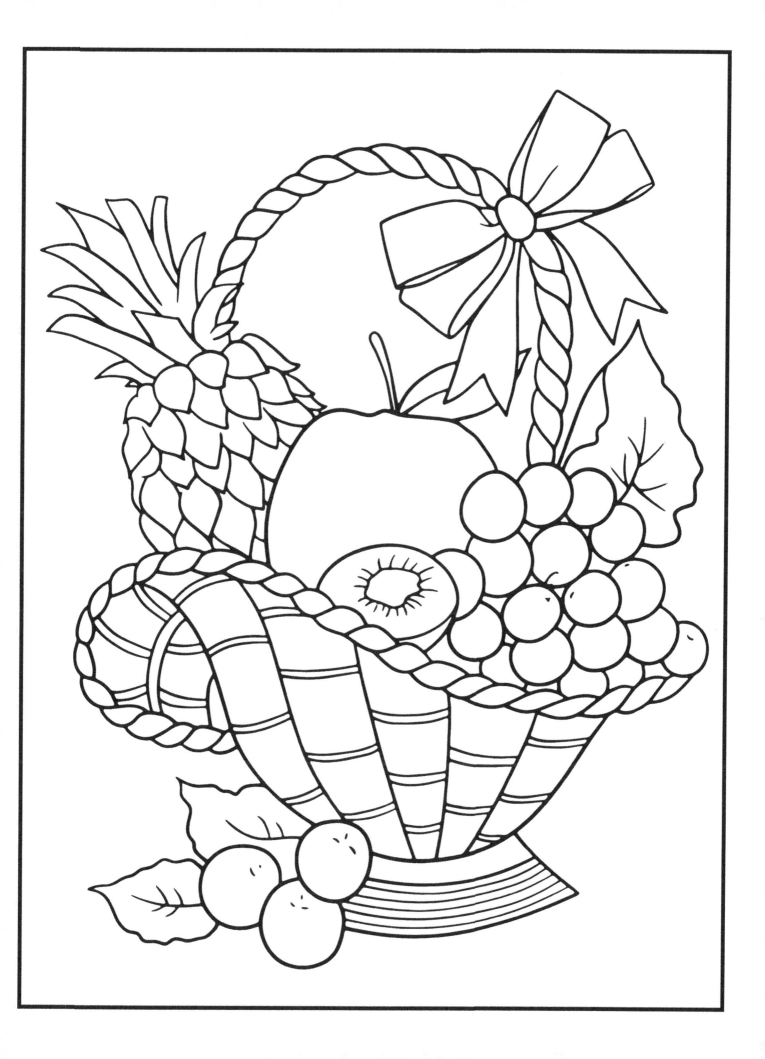

"COLORING IS THE SILENCE THAT SPEAKS WHEN WORDS CAN'T."

- Anonymous

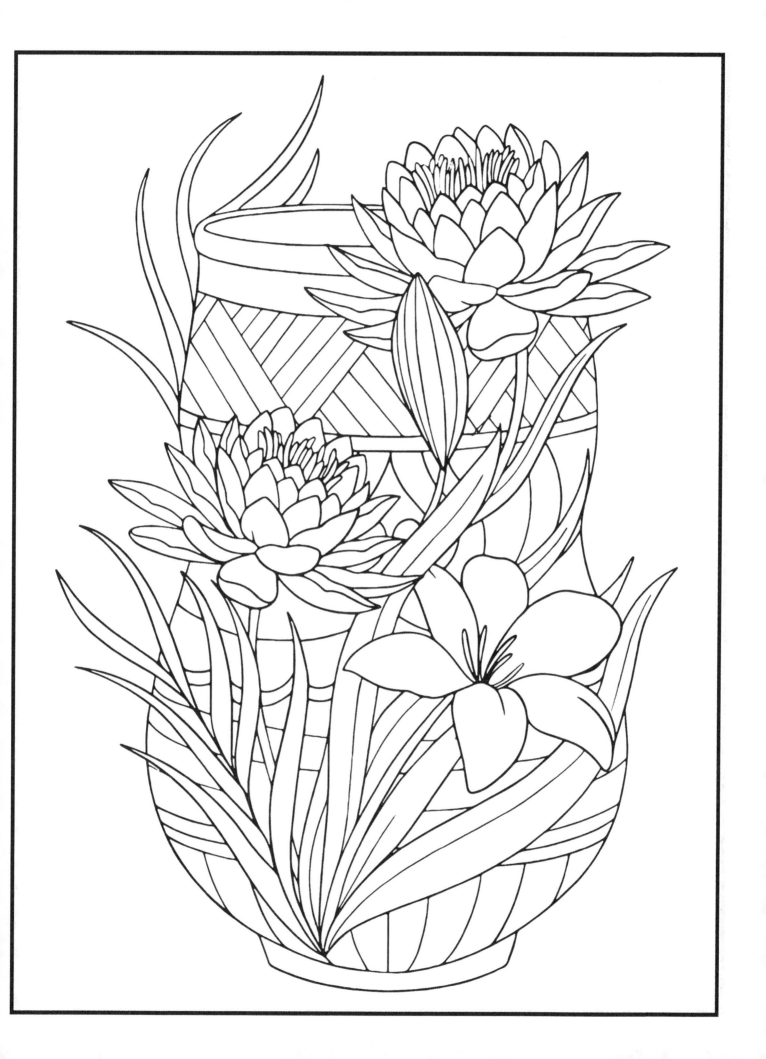

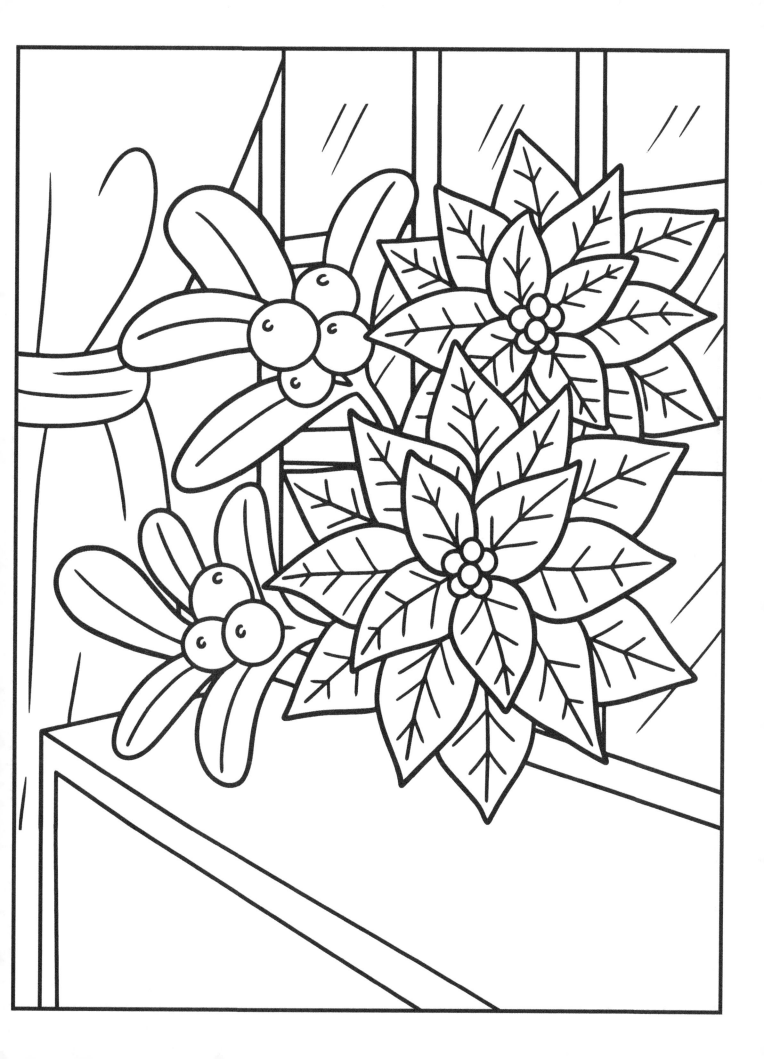

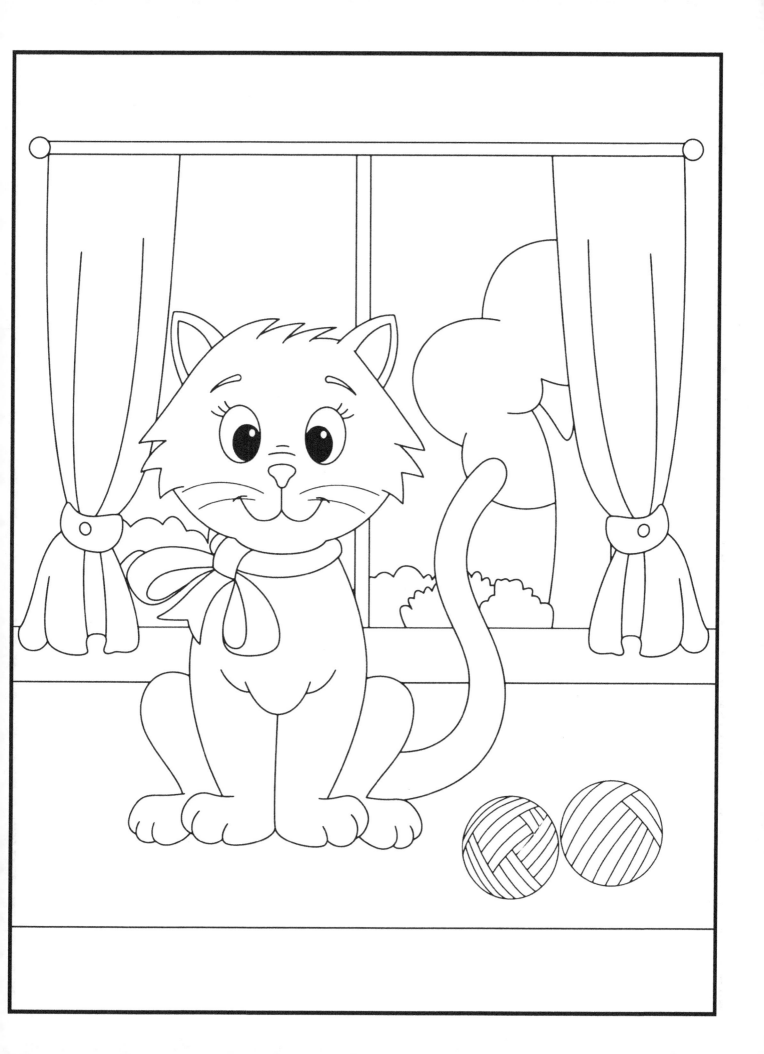

"The world always seems brighter when you've just made something that wasn't there before"

- Neil Gaiman

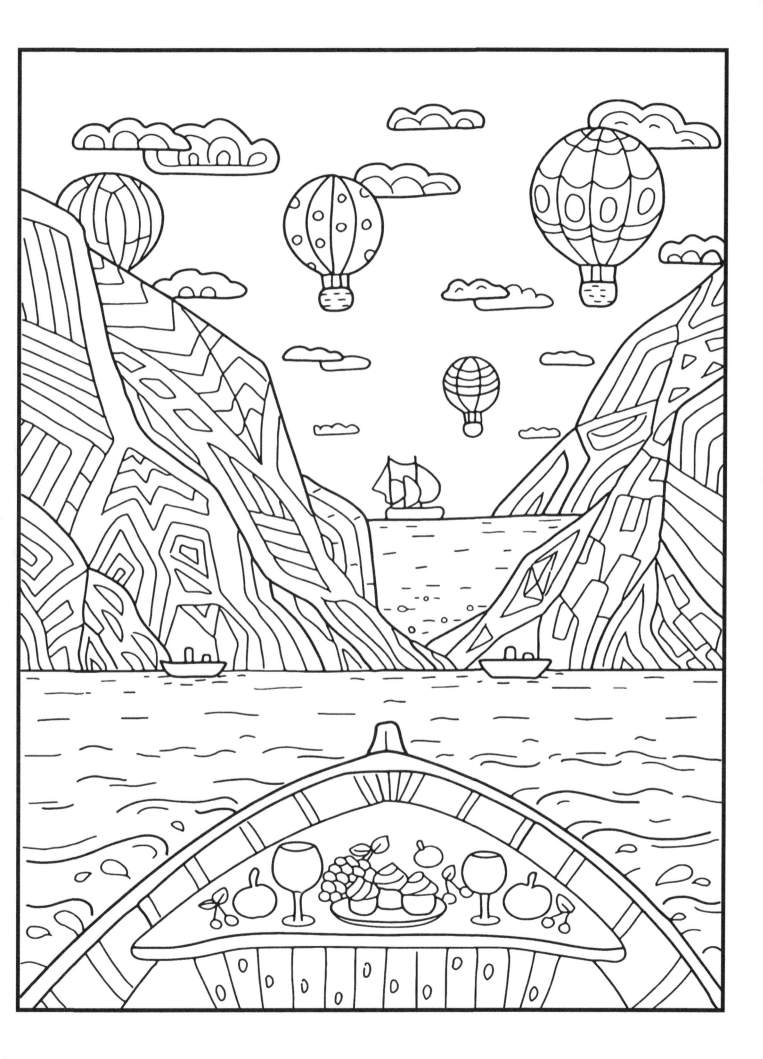

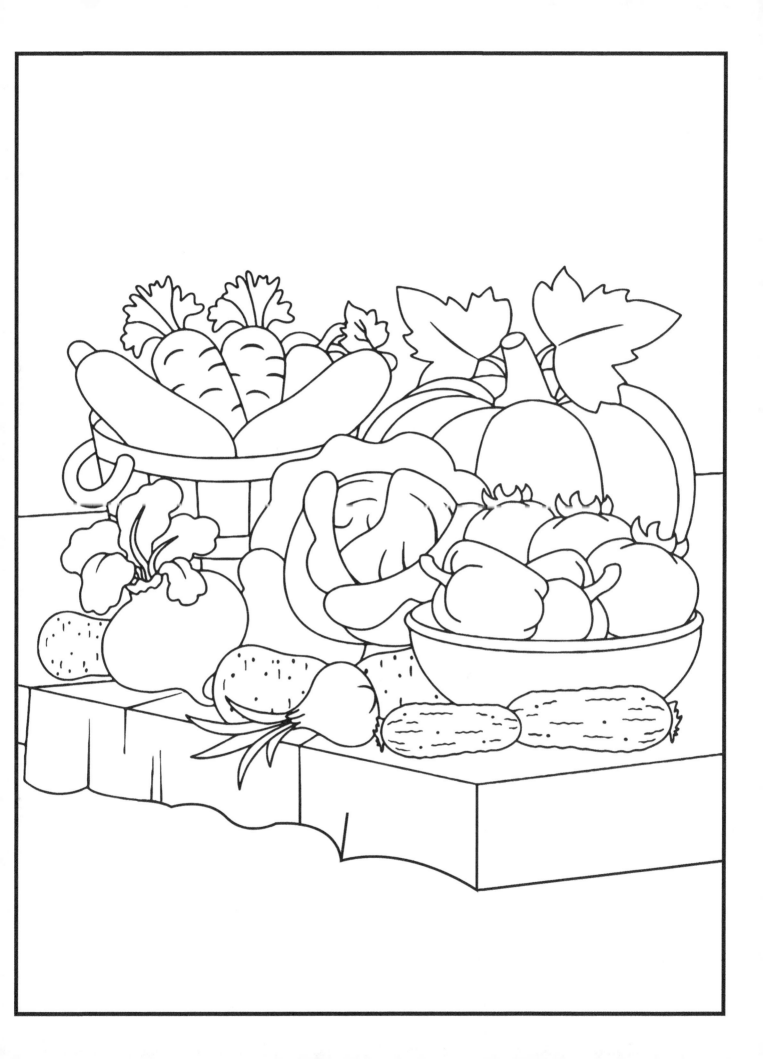

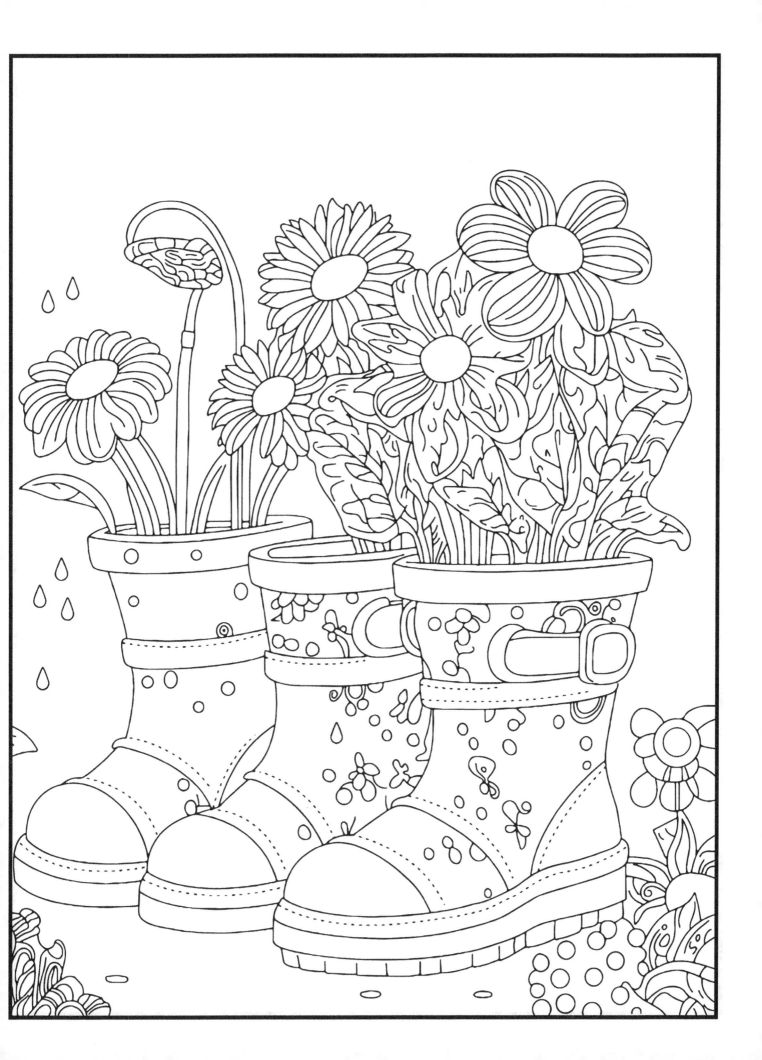

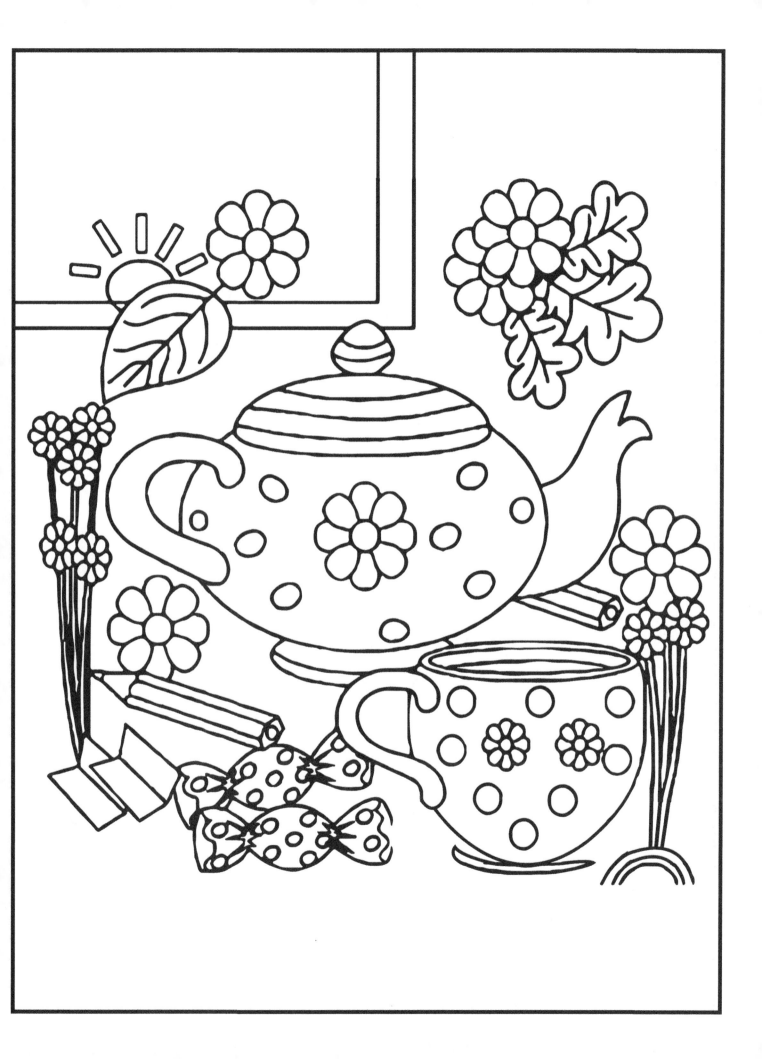

"To live a creative life we must lose our fear of being wrong"

- Joseph Chilton Pearce

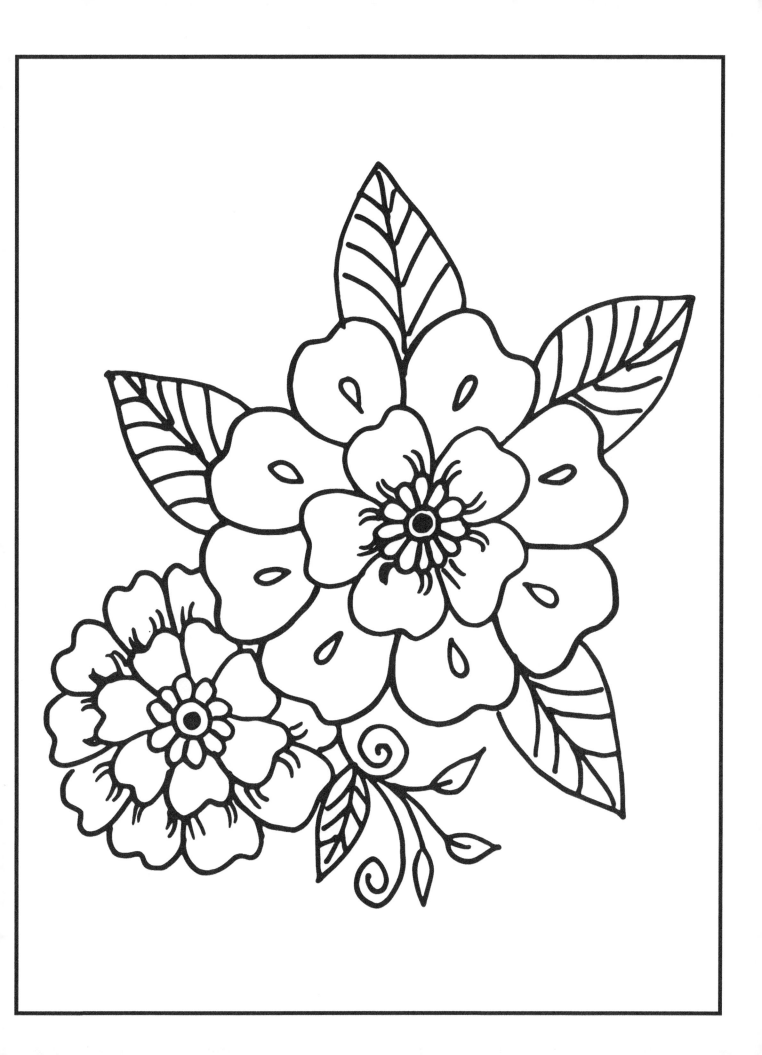

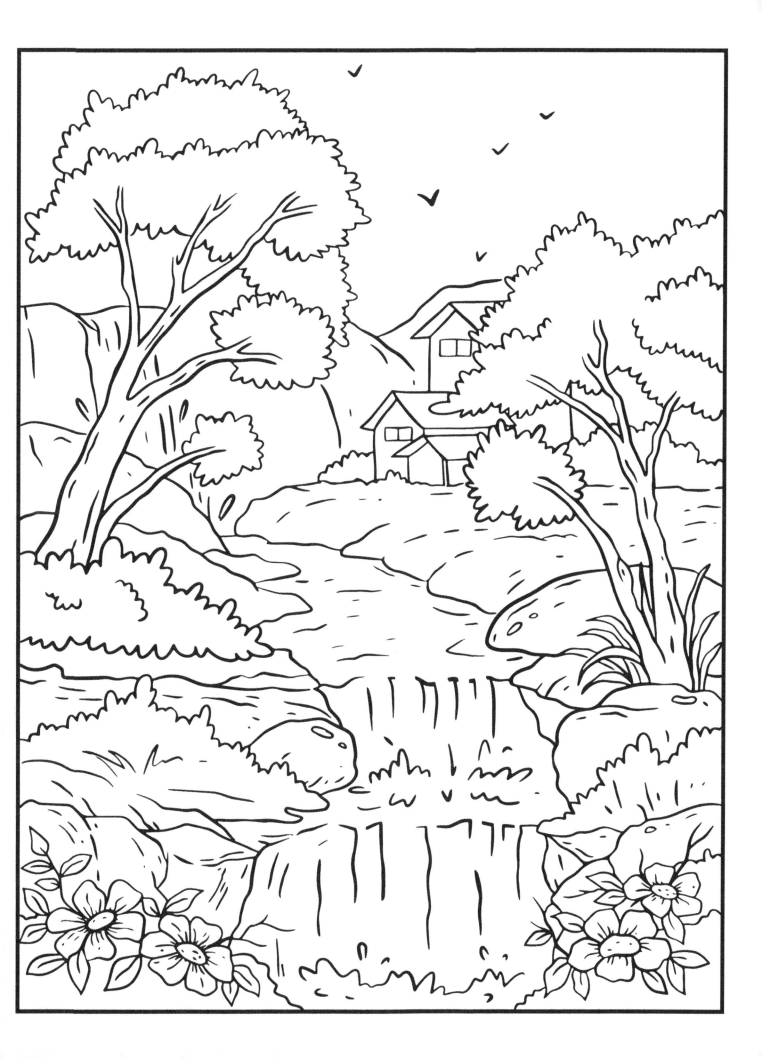

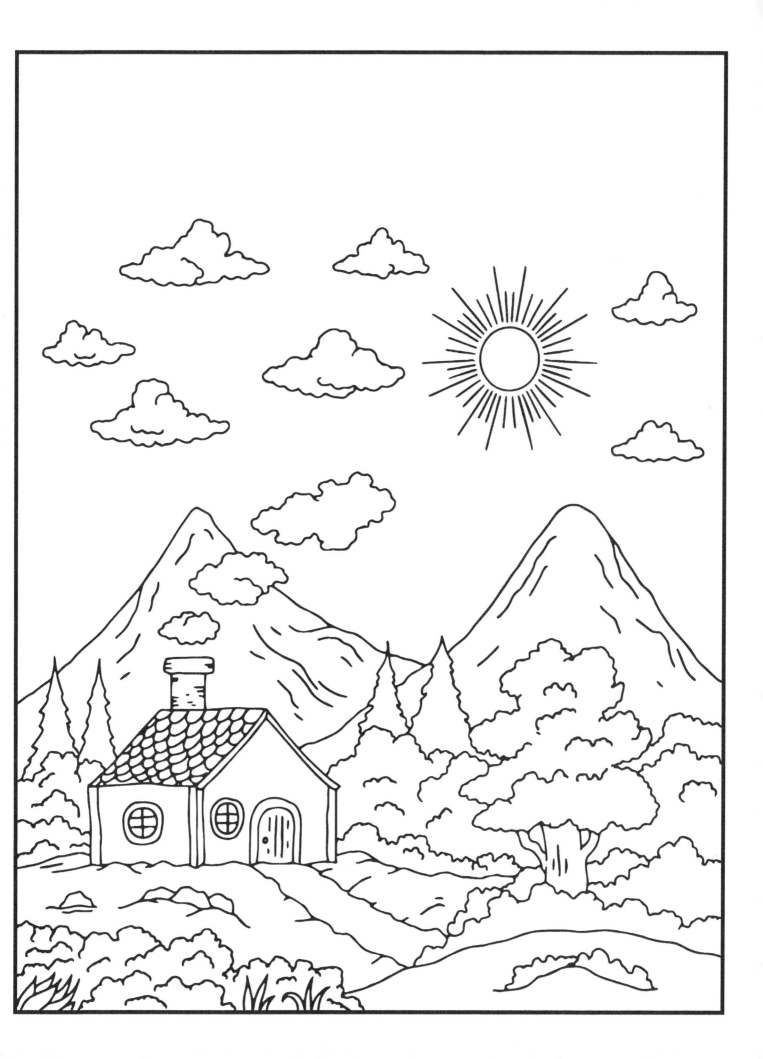

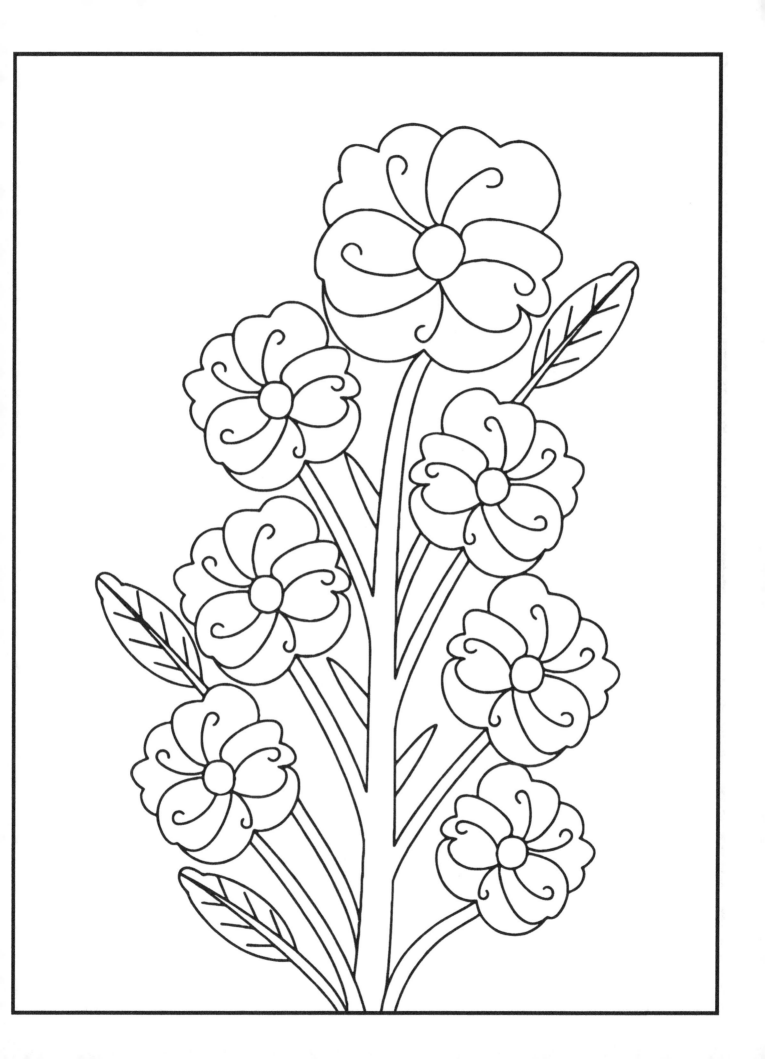

THANK YOU FOR SHARING YOUR ART AT AMAZON

The Benefits of Sharing Your Artwork Online

Scientific studies suggest that sharing your artwork online, such as photos and videos of your beautifully colored pages, can have a significant positive impact on your mental health.

According to a study published in the Journal of Positive Psychology, engaging in creative activities and then sharing them with others can lead to increased feelings of enthusiasm and flourishing. This was found to be true even for those who do not consider themselves 'artists'.

Sharing your creations is believed to boost self-esteem and create a sense of accomplishment. It allows for feedback from others which may help improve skills and foster growth. Plus, it provides an opportunity for social interaction which is known to have numerous psychological benefits.

So there's definitely immense value in sharing your artwork online.

When you take the time to color a page beautifully or create any form of art, don't hesitate to share it on platforms like Amazon checks or social media. Even if you're nervous about how people might react or feel shy about showcasing your talent, remember that the act itself is likely contributing positively towards your mental well-being.

In addition, when you share your work on platforms like Amazon reviews, it also helps other potential buyers get an idea about the product from a user perspective which can be very helpful for them. So not only are you benefiting yourself but also assisting others in their purchasing decisions.

Remember that every piece of art is unique just like its creator and deserves to be shared with the world!

Made in the USA
Middletown, DE
02 July 2025